MIDWIFERY & WOMEN'S HEALTH NURSE PRACTITIONER CERTIFICATION

Study Question Book

Second Edition

Beth M. Kelsey, EdD, WHNP-BC

Assistant Professor
School of Nursing
Ball State University
Muncie, Indiana

Board of Directors
National Association of Nurse Practitioners in Women's Health (NPWH)
Washington, DC

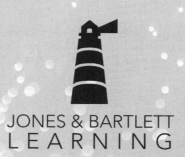

JONES & BARTLETT
LEARNING

World Headquarters
Jones & Bartlett Learning
40 Tall Pine Drive
Sudbury, MA 01776
978-443-5000
info@jblearning.com
www.jblearning.com

Jones & Bartlett Learning
Canada
6339 Ormindale Way
Mississauga, Ontario L5V 1J2
Canada

Jones & Bartlett Learning
International
Barb House, Barb Mews
London W6 7PA
United Kingdom

Jones & Bartlett Learning books and products are available through most bookstores and online booksellers. To contact Jones & Bartlett Learning directly, call 800-832-0034, fax 978-443-8000, or visit our website, www.jblearning.com.

Substantial discounts on bulk quantities of Jones & Bartlett Learning publications are available to corporations, professional associations, and other qualified organizations. For details and specific discount information, contact the special sales department at Jones & Bartlett Learning via the above contact information or send an email to specialsales@jblearning.com.

The author, editor, and publisher have made every effort to provide accurate information. However, they are not responsible for errors, omissions, or for any outcomes related to the use of the contents of this book and take no responsibility for the use of the products and procedures described. Treatments and side effects described in this book may not be applicable to all people; likewise, some people may require a dose or experience a side effect that is not described herein. Drugs and medical devices are discussed that may have limited availability controlled by the Food and Drug Administration (FDA) for use only in a research study or clinical trial. Research, clinical practice, and government regulations often change the accepted standard in this field. When consideration is being given to use of any drug in the clinical setting, the health care provider or reader is responsible for determining FDA status of the drug, reading the package insert, and reviewing prescribing information for the most up-to-date recommendations on dose, precautions, and contraindications, and determining the appropriate usage for the product. This is especially important in the case of drugs that are new or seldom used.

Production Credits

Publisher: Kevin Sullivan
Acquisitions Editor: Amy Sibley
Associate Editor: Patricia Donnelly
Editorial Assistant: Rachel Shuster
Production Editor: Amanda Clerkin
Associate Marketing Manager: Katie Hennessy

V.P., Manufacturing and Inventory Control: Therese Connell
Composition: DataStream Content Solutions, LLC
Cover Design: Kate Ternullo
Cover Image: © Hocusfocus/Dreamstime.com
Printing and Binding: Malloy, Inc.
Cover Printing: Malloy, Inc.

To order this product, use ISBN: 978-1-4496-2970-0

Library of Congress Cataloging-in-Publication Data
Kelsey, Beth.
    Midwifery & women's health nurse practitioner certification study question book / Beth M. Kelsey.   2nd ed.
        p. ; cm.
    Midwifery and women's health nurse practitioner certification study question book
    Rev. ed. of: Midwifery/women's health nurse practitioner certification review guide / editors, Beth M. Kelsey, Patricia Burkardt. c2004.
    Includes bibliographical references and index.
    ISBN 978-0-7637-7743-2
    1. Nurse practitioners—Examinations, questions, etc.   2. Midwives—Examinations, questions, etc.
3. Women—Diseases—Examinations, questions, etc.   4. Women—Health and hygiene—Examinations, questions, etc.   5. Gynecologic nursing—Examinations, questions, etc.   I. Midwifery/women's health nurse practitioner certification review guide.   II. Title.   III. Title: Midwifery and women's health nurse practitioner certification study question book.
    [DNLM: 1. Midwifery—Examination Questions.   2. Genital Diseases, Female—nursing—Examination Questions.   3. Nurse Midwives—Examination Questions.   4. Nurse Practitioners—Examination Questions.
5. Pregnancy Complications—nursing—Examination Questions.   6. Women's Health—Examination Questions.
WY 18.2]
    RT82.8.M53 2012
    610.73092—dc22

2010040549

6048

Printed in the United States of America
15 14 13 12 11   10 9 8 7 6 5 4 3 2 1

Contents

Preface

Jones & Bartlett Learning is pleased to introduce one more component to our complement of nurse practitioner certification review materials. The *Midwifery & Women's Health Nurse Practitioner Certification Study Question Book* will assist the user to be successful in the examination process. It should by no means be the only source used for preparation for the women's health nurse practitioner certification examination. It has been developed primarily to enhance your test-taking skills while also integrating the principles (becoming test-wise) of test taking found in the "Test-Taking Strategies and Skills" chapter of the *Midwifery & Women's Health Nurse Practitioner Certification Review Guide*, also published by Jones & Bartlett Learning. The review guide and the study question book, along with review courses, provide a comprehensive and total approach to success in the examination process. Many individuals feel that taking practice test questions is the most important factor in the certification examination preparation process, yet it is but one strategy to be used in combination with a strong knowledge base. Success in the certification examination area is based upon both excellent test-taking skills and a comprehensive understanding of the content of the

examination. As a nurse practitioner seeking certification, it is important to not lose sight of the definition and purpose of certification. "Certification is the formal recognition of the knowledge, skills, and experience demonstrated by the achievement of standards identified by the profession" (Consensus Model for APRN Regulation: Licensure, Accreditation, Certification, and Education, 2008). Inherent to the preparation for certification examinations is rigorous attention to the directives and materials from the certification boards. Content outlines and sample test questions are often provided to examinees prior to the examinations. Specifics for each examination including suggested readings will be provided by the individual testing boards.

This question book has been prepared by a board certified nurse practitioner. The questions have then been reviewed and critiqued by board certified nurse practitioners (content experts) and a test construction specialist. There are 300 problem-oriented certification board-type multiple choice questions that are divided according to content area (based upon testing board content outlines) with answers, rationales, and a reference list. Every effort has been made to develop sample questions that are representative of the types of questions that may be found on the certification examinations; however, style and format of the examination may differ. Engaging in the exercise of test taking, an understanding of test-taking strategies, and knowledge in respective content areas can only lead to success.

Jones & Bartlett Learning also publishes the *Adult Nurse Practitioner Certification Review Guide, Adult Nurse Practitioner Certification Study Question Book, Pediatric Nurse Practitioner Certification Review Guide*, and *Pediatric Nurse Practitioner Certification Study Question Book*. Family nurse practitioners preparing for their certification examination may find the combination of family, women's health, and pediatric review materials helpful.

The author would like to thank and acknowledge Anne Salomone, MS, RN-C, CNM, for her work on the first edition of this text.

Instructions for Using the Online Access Code Card

Enclosed within this review guide you will find a printed "access code card" containing an access code providing you access to the new online interactive testing program, JB TestPrep. This program will help you prepare for certification exams, such as the American Nurse Credentialing Center's (ANCC's) certification exam to become a certified nurse practitioner. The online program includes the same multiple choice questions that are printed in this study guide. You can choose a "practice exam" that allows you to see feedback on your response immediately, or a "final exam," which hides your results until you have completed all the questions in the exam. Your overall score on the questions you have answered is also compiled. Here are the instructions on how to access JB TestPrep, the Online Interactive Testing Program:

1. Find the printed access code card bound in to this book.
2. Go to www.JBLearning.com/usecode.
3. Enter in your 10-digit access code, which you can find by scratching off the protective coating on the access code card.
4. Follow the instructions on each screen to set up your account profile and password. Please note: Only select a course coordinator if you have been instructed to do so by an institution or an instructor.
5. Contact Jones & Bartlett Learning technical support if you have any questions:
   Call 800-832-0034
   Visit www.jblearning.com and select "Tech Support"
   Email info@jblearning.com

1

Primary Care

Beth M. Kelsey

Anne Salomone

Select one best answer to the following questions.

Questions 1 and 2 refer to the following scenario.

A 66-year-old woman presents to your office for her annual examination in November. She had a mammogram, Pap test, and test for fecal occult blood one year ago. She had a screening sigmoidoscopy 2 years ago. All of these test results were normal. She had her last tetanus-diphtheria (Td) 12 years ago. She had her pneumococcal and influenza vaccinations 1 year ago.

1. Which of the following screening tests should be performed or ordered at this visit?

   a. Mammogram and Pap test
   b. Mammogram and fecal occult blood
   c. Mammogram, Pap test, and sigmoidoscopy
   d. Pap test and fecal occult blood

2. What vaccinations would be recommended at the current visit?

   a. Influenza only
   b. Influenza and pneumococcal
   c. Influenza and Td booster
   d. Influenza, pneumococcal, and Td booster

3. When percussing downward to locate the upper border of the liver, you would expect the percussion tone to change from:

   a. Dullness to flatness
   b. Dullness to resonance
   c. Resonance to dullness
   d. Tympany to dullness

4. When discussing dietary recommendations for prevention of heart disease, you would want to include:

   a. Limit saturated fat intake to no more than 30% of daily calories.
   b. Foods that are low in cholesterol will also be low in fat.
   c. Foods from plant sources do not contain trans fats.
   d. Fish should be consumed at least two times each week.

Questions 5 and 6 refer to the following scenario.

A 30-year-old woman presents to your office to discuss smoking cessation. She currently smokes one pack per day. She tells you she knows she needs to quit but is very concerned about gaining weight. She also tells you that is why she started smoking again 2 years ago after quitting for 6 months.

5. You recognize that she is now in which of the following stages in the process of change?

   a. Action
   b. Contemplation
   c. Precontemplation
   d. Relapse

6. She does decide to try to quit and would like to take bupropion. Information concerning the use of this medication as an aid in smoking cessation would include telling her:

   a. The medication may make it more difficult to keep from gaining weight.
   b. She will need to discontinue smoking for at least 1 week before starting the medication.
   c. She can start the medication on the first day that she does not smoke.
   d. She should wait 1 to 2 weeks after starting the medication before she discontinues smoking.

7. A 22-year-old woman presents to your office with a history suggestive of irritable bowel syndrome. Which of the following symptoms would you expect to be present?

   a. Frequent awakening at night with abdominal cramps
   b. Weight loss related to nausea and loss of appetite
   c. Increase in severity of symptoms with physical activity
   d. Abdominal pain or discomfort relieved with defecation

8. Which of the following pharmacologic treatments for constipation-predominant irritable bowel syndrome is *least* appropriate?

   a. Bulk forming agents
   b. Osmotic laxatives
   c. Stimulant laxatives
   d. Stool softeners

9. A 26-year-old woman presents with abrupt onset diarrhea that started 24 hours ago. She has had approximately six loose stools without any noticeable blood. She has mild abdominal cramping, no nausea, and no fever. Initial management of this patient should include:

   a. Advising liquids rich in electrolytes and sugar
   b. Advising high protein liquid supplements
   c. Obtaining a stool sample for culture
   d. Initiating treatment with antimicrobials

10. A 32-year-old woman presents with a 3-month history of intermittent burning retrosternal pain that radiates to her back. Symptoms are noted 30 to 60 minutes after eating and are relieved quickly by the use of antacids. Physical examination and vital signs are within normal limits (WNL). The most likely diagnosis is:

    a. Acute cholecystitis
    b. Gastric ulcer disease
    c. Gastroesophageal reflux
    d. Ischemic heart disease

11. A 48-year-old female presents with right upper quadrant (RUQ) abdominal pain. As you palpate the RUQ under the costal margin she holds her breath momentarily and reports a sharp increase in the pain. This is most indicative of:

    a. Cholecystitis
    b. Hepatitis
    c. Pancreatitis
    d. Peptic ulcer

Questions 12 and 13 refer to the following scenario.

A 14-year-old sexually active female presents to your office for contraception. She has been having heavy periods since menarche 9 months ago and now has a hemoglobin (Hgb) of 11.0 g/dL. She is otherwise healthy, and her physical examination is normal. She is started on oral contraceptives and ferrous sulfate.

12. One week after starting her iron therapy, the patient calls to tell you that the iron pills make her sick to her stomach and give her heartburn. An appropriate action would be to:

   a. Advise her to take her iron with an antacid
   b. Advise her to take her iron with orange juice
   c. Suggest that she take her iron pills with meals
   d. Switch from oral iron therapy to IM injections

13. Three months later her Hgb is 13.2 g/dL, and her periods are regulated. An appropriate test to determine if her iron stores have been replenished is a:

   a. Total iron binding capacity
   b. Plasma transferrin level
   c. Reticulocyte count
   d. Serum ferritin level

14. An African-American couple planning a pregnancy presents to your office with questions about sickle cell anemia. Both of them carry the sickle cell trait. The likelihood that their child will have sickle cell disease is:

   a. 0%
   b. 25%
   c. 50%
   d. 100%

15. The definitive test for sickle cell anemia is the:

   a. Hgb electrophoresis
   b. Indirect Coombs
   c. Sickledex preparation
   d. Schilling test

Questions 16, 17, and 18 refer to the following scenario.

When taking a health history on a 35-year-old woman, you learn that she has a history of migraine headaches. She tells you that in the last year they have occurred two to three times each month. She takes over-the-counter pain medication and has to go to bed when she has the headaches.

16. Which of the following characteristics is *not* typically associated with migraine headaches?

   a. The headache is often accompanied by nausea.
   b. The age of onset is usually > 30.
   c. The headaches can last for up to 72 hours.
   d. The location of the pain is usually unilateral.

17. Because this patient's headaches are occurring two or more times each month, preventive therapy is being considered. Which of the following medications is indicated for preventive therapy of migraine headaches?

   a. Beta-adrenergic blocking agents
   b. Codeine containing analgesics
   c. Ergotamine preparations
   d. Sumatriptan

18. If sumatriptan is prescribed, the client should be instructed that:

   a. This medication should be taken at the onset of a headache before taking any other pain medications.
   b. The effectiveness of this medication can be improved when combined with an ergotamine.
   c. A common side-effect of this medication is nausea and vomiting.
   d. This medication should be used with caution due to its addictive potential.

Questions 19 and 20 refer to the following scenario.

A 30-year-old female who does repetitive small parts work in a factory presents with the complaint of intermittent numbness and tingling in the fingers of her right hand.

19. Physical examination reveals a positive Tinel's sign and a positive Phalen's maneuver. These two tests are usually positive with:

    a. Multiple sclerosis
    b. Raynaud's phenomenon
    c. Carpal tunnel syndrome
    d. Stress fractures of the wrist

20. Considering the patient's symptoms and the two positive tests, what other findings would you expect?

    a. Blanching of the fingers when cold
    b. Excess sweating of the hand palms
    c. Neck pain that radiates down the arm
    d. Increase in symptoms during the night

21. A 40-year-old female presents with gradual onset of sharp, shooting lower back pain that radiates to the left thigh and lower leg. She has limited active flexion and extension of the back due to pain. She has a positive straight leg raise test. The most likely diagnosis is:

    a. Ankylosing spondylitis
    b. Herniated intervertebral disk
    c. Lumbosacral strain
    d. Spinal stenosis

22. The patient with low back pain related to lumbosacral strain should be advised that:

    a. Abdominal strengthening exercises help to prevent recurrence.
    b. Heat therapy, rather than cold packs, should be used for pain relief.
    c. One to two weeks of bedrest may be necessary for full recovery.
    d. Back stretching exercises are an important part of therapy.

23. Which of the following history or physical examination findings is characteristic of osteoarthritis?

    a. Crepitus upon movement of the affected joints
    b. Joint pain that gets worse as the day progresses
    c. Soft tissue swelling around the affected joints
    d. Presence of fatigue and general malaise

24. A 34-year-old female presents with complaints of fatigue and generalized muscle and joint pain for the past several months. She has normal range of motion, no apparent swelling of joints, and no abnormal neurologic findings. She has multiple tender points over the muscles on both sides of her body when pressure is applied. A probable diagnosis is:

    a. Fibromyalgia
    b. Lupus erythematosus
    c. Polymyalgia rheumatica
    d. Rheumatoid arthritis

Questions 25 and 26 refer to the following scenario.

A 32-year-old female presents with a recent onset of irregular patches of erythema and oozing vesicles on her hands. She complains of itching and burning of the affected areas.

25. The most likely cause for her symptoms is:

    a. Contact dermatitis
    b. Fungal infection
    c. Cellulitis
    d. Scabies

26. Appropriate treatment for this condition is:

    a. Erythromycin
    b. Ketoconazole
    c. Permethrin 5% cream
    d. Topical corticosteroids

27. A 25-year-old female presents in your office for her annual examination. You notice a 5 cm annular lesion with a pale center on her leg. She states it does not itch and that she first noticed it about 1 week after returning from a camping trip she took last month. A likely diagnosis is:

    a. Cellulitis
    b. Lyme disease
    c. Poison ivy
    d. Spider bite

28. An ulcerated nodule with a translucent surface and firm raised borders on the face is most likely:

    a. Actinic keratosis
    b. Basal cell carcinoma
    c. Herpes zoster
    d. Squamous cell carcinoma

29. A 58-year-old female presents with new onset unilateral throbbing headache along with scalp tenderness. She also complains of jaw pain, anorexia, and fatigue. Her temperature is 101°F. Appropriate initial management would include ordering:

    a. CT scan
    b. Erythrocyte sedimentation rate
    c. Lumbar puncture
    d. Sinus radiographs

30. A 22-year-old female presents with the complaint that for the past 24 hours her right eye has felt "scratchy" and had a watery discharge. She reports no problems with vision and no photophobia. Examination reveals peripheral injection with watery discharge in the right eye. A likely cause for her symptoms is:

    a. Allergic conjunctivitis
    b. Corneal abrasion
    c. Subconjunctival hemorrhage
    d. Viral conjunctivitis

Questions 31 and 32 refer to the following scenario.

A 27-year-old woman confides in you that her husband has been both emotionally and physically abusive to her over the past several years. She says that since the last abuse 2 weeks ago, he has actually been very attentive and has promised to quit drinking.

31. An appropriate initial plan of care for this woman would include encouragement to:

    a. Discuss the abuse that has occurred in specific and concrete terms
    b. Discuss what she has done differently in the past 2 weeks
    c. Leave the situation immediately and seek legal recourse
    d. Talk with her partner about seeing a counselor as a couple

32. In relation to the cycle of violence, you could describe to the woman how her husband's current behavior is typical of the:

    a. Tension building phase
    b. Recovery phase
    c. Honeymoon phase
    d. Reality phase

33. A 30-year-old woman comes to your office for follow-up of minor injuries sustained in a car accident. She admits that she was arrested for driving under the influence of alcohol, and that her husband has moved out because of her drinking. She states that she did quit drinking for a few days after the accident, but felt like she was going to crawl out of her skin. Which of the following pieces of information would indicate that she has an alcohol dependency?

    a. She drinks in situations in which alcohol use is physically hazardous.
    b. She has interpersonal problems related to her alcohol use.

c. She has repeated legal problems directly related to alcohol use.

d. She makes unsuccessful attempts to cut down or control alcohol use.

34. A physical sign suggestive of moderate-to-severe insulin resistance is:

a. Butterfly rash on malar area of face
b. Hirsutism on face and upper body
c. Hyperpigmented, velvety thickening of skin on neck and axilla
d. Spider angiomas on face, abdomen, and lower extremities

35. All of the following are characteristic symptoms of interstitial cystitis *except*:

a. Bladder pain that decreases with voiding
b. Pain with sexual intercourse
c. Persistent urge to void
d. Urinary incontinence

36. Similarities between the two eating disorders of anorexia nervosa and bulimia include:

a. Substance abuse as an accompanying problem
b. Amenorrhea as part of the diagnostic criteria
c. Lack of control as a predominating feature
d. Depression often accompanying the eating disorder

Questions 37 and 38 refer to the following scenario.

A 35-year-old female has been diagnosed with major depression. She states that she has had several symptoms of depression for the past month including loss of appetite, insomnia, loss of energy, and inability to concentrate.

37. To meet the DSM-IV diagnostic criteria for major depression, she must also exhibit:

a. Feelings of worthlessness or excessive guilt
b. Thoughts about dying or committing suicide

c. Loss of interest or pleasure in most activities
d. Previous occurrence of the same symptoms

38. Her primary care provider has prescribed trazodone (a heterocyclic antidepressant), and paroxetine (a serotonin reuptake inhibitor), as part of her treatment. Client education should include instructing her that:

a. They should be taken on alternating days to avoid an overdose.
b. They should both be taken at night for optimal effect.
c. She should try both separately and decide which is most helpful.
d. Paroxetine should be taken in the morning and trazodone at night.

39. In relation to the current leading cause of death in children and adolescents, one of the most important topics for anticipatory guidance for a 16-year-old female would include discussion about:

a. Always wearing seat belts in the car
b. Annual Pap tests if she is sexually active
c. Monthly self-breast examination
d. Condom use and abstinence

40. Which of the following is an American Diabetes Association (ADA) recommended goal for reduction of cardiovascular disease in the individual with diabetes mellitus?

a. Maintain blood pressure at less than 140/90
b. Maintain LDL cholesterol of less than 100 mg/dL
c. Maintain an HbA1c at less than 8%
d. Maintain saturated fat intake to less than 15% of total calories

41. When conducting the Weber test on an individual with hearing loss related to obstruction of the ear canal with excessive cerumen in the left ear, you would expect:

a. Air conduction longer than bone conduction in the left ear

b. Bone conduction longer than air conduction in the left ear
c. Sound heard better in the left ear
d. Sound heard better in the right ear

42. Asking the patient to clench her teeth while you palpate the temporal and masseter muscles is a test for which cranial nerve?

a. CN IV Trochlear
b. CN V Trigeminal
c. CN VI Abducens
d. CN VII Facial

43. A friction rub is most likely to be heard with:

a. Mitral stenosis
b. Pericarditis
c. Pneumonia
d. Pneumothorax

44. A 50-year-old female presents with complaint of severe pleuritic chest pain and dyspnea that started a few hours ago. She returned from a trip to Europe 1 week ago and felt fine until today. Physical examination reveals temperature of 100.2°F, respirations 24, shallow and labored, and heart rate 98 bpm with regular rate and rhythm. She has diminished breath sounds, and you note dullness to percussion in the left lower lobe. The most likely diagnosis is:

a. Acute myocardial infarction
b. Pericarditis
c. Pneumothorax
d. Pulmonary embolism

45. A 22-year-old female presents with complaints of intermittent palpitations and occasional chest pain that she describes as sharp and not related to exertion. She is 5 ft. 2 in., 106 lbs., and has normal vital signs. Her physical examination is normal except for a midsystolic click and a systolic murmur. The most useful test to confirm her likely diagnosis would be a/an:

a. Chest radiograph
b. Cardiac enzyme panel

c. Echocardiogram
d. Electrocardiogram

46. Which of the following physical examination findings would correlate with an elevated TSH and a suppressed FT_4 level?

a. Exophthalmos
b. Nystagmus
c. Periorbital edema
d. Ptosis of the eyelids

47. The usual sequence of female pubertal events is:

a. Breast development, growth of pubic and axillary hair, menses, peak increase in height
b. Breast development, growth of pubic and axillary hair, peak increase in height, menses
c. Peak increase in height, breast development, menses, growth of pubic and axillary hair
d. Growth of pubic and axillary hair, peak increase in height, breast development, menses

48. A 20-year-old female presents with sore throat, nasal stuffiness, cough, and general malaise for the past 2 days. Physical examination reveals mild pharyngeal erythema with no exudate, negative lymphadenopathy, and temperature of 99.8°F. Appropriate initial management would include:

a. Obtain pharyngeal culture and initiate antibiotics while awaiting results
b. Obtain rapid strep screen, if negative do culture and await results to determine if needs antibiotics
c. Obtain rapid strep screen, if negative, do not do culture or treat with antibiotics
d. Treat with antibiotics on basis of risk factors for streptococcal pharyngitis

49. Which of the following sections of the client's record should include only objective information?

a. History of present illness
b. Physical examination
c. Problem list
d. Review of systems

50. A 35-year-old female presents with a complaint of nervousness, increased perspiration, weight loss despite an increased appetite, and frequent bowel movements. Abnormal examination findings include patellar reflexes 3+, heart rate 100 bpm, and a moderately enlarged, soft, nontender thyroid gland. The most likely diagnosis is:

a. Graves' disease
b. Hypothyroidism
c. Myxedema
d. Thyroiditis

51. Which of the following individuals does *not* need further evaluation with a fasting lipid profile?

a. 58-year-old female with total cholesterol 210, HDL 40, no other risk factors
b. 30-year-old female with total cholesterol 190, HDL 45, smoker; no other risk factors
c. 26-year-old female with total cholesterol 200, HDL 35, smoker; no other risk factors
d. 40-year-old female with total cholesterol 200, HDL 35, no other risk factors

52. A 60-year-old female presents with pleuritic chest pain and a cough productive of yellow sputum. Her temperature is 101°F, respirations 32, and heart rate 90 bpm. She appears to be somewhat dehydrated. Expected findings on physical examination would include:

a. Decreased vocal fremitus
b. Jugular venous distention
c. Areas of dullness over lungs
d. Absence of bronchophony

53. Which of the following is true concerning the use of fecal occult blood testing for colon cancer screening?

a. This screening test can be done with a sample obtained during digital rectal examination.
b. This screening should be done annually starting at 40 years of age.
c. A positive test should be followed with repeat testing in 1 month.
d. The individual should avoid vitamin C and citrus fruits for several days before the test.

54. According to the CDC criteria for preventive therapy of tuberculosis, an individual with a PPD test showing an induration of 5 mm or greater would meet the criteria for having a positive skin test if she:

a. Is foreign born from a country with high TB prevalence
b. Has had close contact with an individual who has active TB infection
c. Is an intravenous drug user
d. Previously received a BCG vaccination

55. Antinuclear antibody (ANA) tests are most likely to be positive in:

a. Acute gouty arthritis
b. Fibromyalgia
c. Osteoarthritis
d. Rheumatoid arthritis

56. Management of systemic lupus erythematosus includes:

a. Avoidance of all hormonal contraception
b. Obtaining autoantibody tests every 6 months
c. Regular exposure to ultraviolet light
d. Use of corticosteroids

57. Which of the following statements is true concerning Rapid HIV screening tests?

a. Sensitivity and specificity are comparable with traditional tests sent to a laboratory.
b. Positive results are definitive so a second test for confirmation is not needed.

   c. It may take longer after exposure to HIV for rapid test to be positive compared with traditional tests sent to laboratory.

   d. Rapid HIV tests have not been FDA approved.

58. The presence of hepatitis B surface antibody (HBsAb) indicates:

   a. Active hepatitis B infection
   b. Carrier state for hepatitis B infection
   c. Early convalescent stage of hepatitis B infection
   d. Immunity to hepatitis B infection

59. A 33-year-old female recently saw a show on chronic fatigue syndrome. She tells you that she thinks she may have this condition because she has been extremely fatigued for the past month and has had pain in her joints. In evaluating this client you will want to take into consideration that:

   a. A diagnosis of chronic fatigue syndrome requires that symptoms persist for at least 3 months.
   b. Symptoms commonly include sore throat, headaches, and both joint and muscle pain.
   c. This condition occurs most frequently during the perimenopause and is likely hormone related.
   d. Physical findings commonly include joint inflammation, muscle weakness, and generalized lymphadenopathy.

60. Evidence-based treatment for chronic fatigue syndrome includes:

   a. Multivitamin supplementation
   b. Moderate aerobic exercise program
   c. Initiation of a low-dose SSRI
   d. Initiation of systemic corticosteroids

◻ ANSWERS AND RATIONALE

1. **(b)** The American Cancer Society (ACS) provides the following cancer screening recommendations: Women age 40 and older should have annual mammograms continuing for as long as the woman is in good health. Beginning at age 30, women who have had three normal Pap test results in a row may get screened every 2 to 3 years or may have Pap test with HPV test every 3 years. Fecal occult blood testing (FOBT) or fecal immunochemical test (FIT) should be conducted annually starting at age 50. Sigmoidoscopy should be conducted every 5 years or colonoscopy every 10 years or double-contrast barium enema every 5 years or CT colonography (virtual colonoscopy) every 5 years starting at age 50 (Smith et al, pp. 161–163, 165–167).

2. **(c)** The Centers for Disease Control and Prevention (CDC) Advisory Committee on Immunization Practices makes the following immunization recommendations that would apply to the 65-year-old woman in this question: Influenza immunization should be given annually; all immunocompetent individuals age 65 and older should be immunized once with pneumococcal vaccine (one-time revaccination is recommended if vaccinated ≥ 5 years previously and aged < 65 years at the time of primary vaccination); and adults should receive a tetanus-diphtheria (Td) booster vaccination every 10 years. A herpes zoster vaccination is also recommended for individuals age 60 and older (CDC, pp. 1–2).

3. **(c)** The sound heard when percussing downward in the midclavicular line to find the upper border of the liver will change from resonance when over the lung fields to dull when over the liver (Bickley, p. 439).

4. **(d)** The American Heart Association (AHA) recommends that total fat be limited to 25 to 35%, saturated fats to less than 7%, and trans fats to less than 1% of daily caloric intake. Trans fats are found in products that contain partially hydrogenated fat as well as in meat and whole-fat dairy products. Replacing meats with vegetable alternatives (e.g.,

beans) or fish is one strategy to replace saturated fats with unsaturated fats and reduce the cholesterol content. A food can be low in cholesterol yet still be high in saturated fat. An example is peanut butter. Fish, especially oily fish, should be consumed at least two times each week. Fish is low in saturated fat and trans fats and contains omega-3 polyunsaturated fatty acids associated with a decreased risk of cardiovascular disease (Lichtenstein et al., pp. 87–88).

5. **(b)** The Transtheoretical Model for Change (DiClemente & Prochaska) has five stages: precontemplation, contemplation, action, maintenance/relapse prevention, and relapse. The individual who expresses an awareness that the current behavior is a problem is in the contemplation stage. The healthcare provider can help the individual by discussing her reasons for wanting to change, risks of not making a change, and any barriers about which she is concerned (Buttaro et al., pp. 133–134; Hackley et al., pp. 230–233).

6. **(d)** Bupropion is an antidepressant found to be helpful in smoking cessation. This is likely due to its effect on the neural uptake of dopamine, prolonging the action of this neurotransmitter. Weight gain is not a side-effect of this medication. It is recommended to start bupropion 1 to 2 weeks before the smoking quit date so blood levels of the medication will be stabilized. Bupropion is contraindicated for individuals with seizure disorders and eating disorders (Buttaro et al., p. 136).

7. **(d)** Criteria for the diagnosis of irritable bowel syndrome (IBS) include continuous or recurrent symptoms, for at least 3 months, of abdominal pain or discomfort relieved with defecation or associated with a change in frequency or consistency of stool. The individual must also have an irregular pattern of defecation at least 25% of the time with three or more of the following:

altered stool frequency, altered stool form, altered stool passage, passage of mucus and bloating, or feeling of abdominal distention. Typically IBS does not awaken the individual nor does it result in significant weight loss. Physical activity generally does not cause an increase in severity of symptoms and regular physical exercise may benefit the individual with IBS (Buttaro et al., pp. 693–695).

8. **(c)** Increasing dietary fiber will result in a bulkier stool and is considered appropriate treatment for both diarrhea and constipation in IBS. Bulk forming agents such as psyllium husk fiber and methylcellulose can also be used for this purpose. Although regular use of laxatives is not recommended, individuals with constipation-predominant IBS may use stool softeners and osmotic laxatives as needed. Stimulant laxatives should be avoided as much as possible (Buttaro et al., p. 697; Ferri, pp. 535–536).

9. **(a)** Acute diarrhea is usually self-limiting. Food should be restricted, but oral hydration should be maintained with fluids rich in electrolytes. Restart foods slowly as tolerated with clear liquids and then carbohydrates. Resume protein and fats last. Stool culture may be indicated if symptoms persist and/or if the client has fever or bloody stools (Buttaro et al., pp. 654–657).

10. **(c)** The intermittent nature, location, and timing of the pain, along with its association of relief with antacids, is highly suggestive of gastroesophageal reflux disease (GERD). If there is suspicion of heart disease or other disorders, appropriate evaluation is indicated (Buttaro et al., pp. 666–667; Dains et al., p. 187).

11. **(a)** The pain of cholecystitis is usually colicky, constant, and located in the right upper quadrant of the abdomen. Deep inspiration usually causes severe

pain and splitting of respiration (holding breath). This is known as Murphy's sign (Dains et al., pp. 184–185).

12. **(c)** Approximately 15 to 20% of individuals experience gastrointestinal side-effects with oral iron supplementation. While iron is better absorbed on an empty stomach, ingesting it with food may decrease gastric irritation so that the individual will continue to take the iron. Other options would be to try a different iron preparation or to slowly increase dosage. While vitamin C increases absorption, taking her iron with orange juice will probably not alleviate gastric irritation. Antacids inhibit absorption. IM iron injections are usually not required (Buttaro et al., p. 1186; Hackley et al., pp. 543–544).

13. **(d)** Serum ferritin is the major iron storage protein. It is present in serum concentrations directly related to iron stores (Hackley et al., p. 541).

14. **(b)** If both parents are carriers of the sickle cell trait, they each have one affected gene and one normal gene for the disorder. Each offspring has a 25% chance of receiving the affected gene from both parents. In an autosomal recessive disorder both genes must be affected for the individual to have the disease (Buttaro et al., p. 1188).

15. **(a)** Hgb electrophoresis is the test of choice for distinguishing between the carrier and the affected state. It is very accurate in identifying the types of hemoglobin in a blood sample. Sickledex preparation is a commonly used screening test. A positive Sickledex must be confirmed with Hgb electrophoresis (Buttaro et al., p. 1194).

16. **(b)** Migraine headaches usually begin in adolescence or early adulthood, although they can occur in young children. Migraine headaches are typically unilateral and throbbing, can last up to 72 hours, and are often accompanied by nausea and photophobia (Buttaro et al., pp. 1052–1053; Dains et al., pp. 403, 406).

17. **(a)** Beta-adrenergic blocking agents such as propranolol are indicated for preventive therapy of migraine headache. The other three medications are indicated for abortive or analgesic therapy of acute migraine headaches (Buttaro et al., pp. 1057–1058; Ferri p. 374).

18. **(a)** Sumatriptan should be taken at the onset of a headache for best results. It has the beneficial effect of also helping to relieve nausea. It should not be used if ergotamine preparations have been used in the past 24 hours. Sumatriptan is not considered to carry a risk for addiction (Wynne et al., pp. 995–996).

19. **(c)** Carpal tunnel syndrome is caused by compression or irritation of the median nerve at the wrist. Often there is no apparent predisposing cause, but overuse activities with repetitive flexion at the wrist or pincer motion may precipitate this syndrome. Typical symptoms include a dull aching pain across the wrist and forearm with paresthesia, weakness, or clumsiness of the hand. Tinel's sign is elicited by tapping over the median nerve at the palmar surface of the wrist. Tinel's sign is positive when the client has a tingling or prickling sensation along the first three digits, wrist pain, and weak grip. Phalen's sign is positive when the client experiences numbness and paraesthesia in the fingers innervated by the median nerve after maintaining palmar flexion for 1 minute. These are both seen with carpal tunnel syndrome (Dains et al., pp. 370–371).

20. **(d)** Nocturnal pain and radiation of pain up to the proximal forearm are also common symptoms with carpal tunnel syndrome. Examination findings—in addition to positive Tinel's and Phalen's signs—may include muscle

atrophy and dry skin on the affected hand (Dains et al., pp. 370, 375).

21. **(b)** Symptoms associated with a herniated intravertebral disk (the most common cause of sciatica) include low back pain and burning that radiates along the lateral thigh, leg, and foot. Physical examination findings include pain below the knee with elevation of the affected leg with patient in sitting or supine position (positive straight leg raise). This pain may also be felt in the buttocks and posterior thigh (Buttaro et al., pp. 976–978; Dains et al., p. 385).

22. **(a)** Abdominal strengthening exercises are useful in preventing recurrence of lumbosacral back strain. The use of heat, cold packs, or the combination of both can be useful in providing relief of this type of back pain. Bedrest should be limited to 2–3 days. Back stretching exercises have been shown to be of little value and are not recommended (Buttaro et al., p. 978).

23. **(a)** Osteoarthritis is a degenerative disease of the cartilage of joints. It is the most common form of chronic arthritis, affecting up to 25% of the adult population. Common presenting history is asymmetrical joint pain and stiffness that improves throughout the day. Joints involved typically include the distal and proximal interphalangeal joints, hips, knees, and the cervical and lumbar spine. Physical examination findings typically include crepitus and limited range of motion of the joints. The joints feel cool with bony enlargement. Constitutional signs such as fatigue and malaise are not characteristic of osteoarthritis (Dains et al, pp. 363, 372).

24. **(a)** Fibromyalgia is characterized by unexplained widespread pain or aching, persistent fatigue, generalized morning stiffness, nonrefreshing sleep and multiple tender points. Pain over specific point sites can be elicited with digital pressure over these areas. Findings are bilateral and involve both the upper and lower body. Changes in range of motion, swelling in the joints, and abnormal neurologic findings are not characteristic of fibromyalgia (Buttaro et al., pp. 948–950).

25. **(a)** Contact dermatitis is characterized by pruritus or burning at the site of contact of an irritant or allergen. Lesions vary depending on the stage of response. In the acute stage erythema and oozing vesicles are common. Fungal infection typically affects scalp, trunk, limbs, face, groin, or feet and is characterized by erythematous, scaling plaques. Cellulitis is characterized by diffuse, sharply defined erythema. Red streaks run from the cellulitis toward regional lymph nodes. Scabies is characterized by minute vesicles and linear runs or burrows often found in digital webs, palms, wrists, gluteal folds, buttocks, and toes (Buttaro et al., pp. 245, 247, 260–261, 287; Dains et al., pp. 93–94).

26. **(d)** Topical corticosteroid agents are generally effective in the treatment of mild, uncomplicated contact dermatitis. Systemic corticosteroid therapy may be indicated for more severe episodes (Buttaro et al., p. 248).

27. **(b)** The characteristic lesion of Lyme disease (erythema migrans) is annular and erythematous with central pallor at the site of the tick bite. The lesion usually starts at about 5 cm in diameter and grows rapidly to about 20 cm. It typically appears within 1 week to 1 month after the tick bite and is nonpruritic. The patient may begin to have constitutional symptoms such as fatigue, myalgias, arthralgias, headache, and fever during the localized phase that extend to symptoms of involvement of other organ systems if not treated early (Buttaro et al., pp. 1330–1331).

28. **(d)** Squamous cell carcinoma presents on sun-exposed surfaces such as the face. The lesion starts as a firm nodule or papule with thick scale that becomes eroded, crusted, and ulcerated with raised pearly borders. Basal cell carcinoma usually appears on the head, neck or hands as a small nodule that if untreated will begin to bleed and crust over. Characteristics of malignant melanoma include: A—asymmetry of borders, B—border irregularity or notching, C—color variation, and D—diameter greater than 6 mm. Malignant melanoma is seen in young, middle-aged, and older adults (Dains et al., pp. 94–95, 99).

29. **(b)** Temporal arteritis presents as sharp, throbbing, or aching pain localized to the temporal area. Other symptoms may include scalp tenderness, jaw pain with chewing, anorexia, weight loss, and fatigue. The individual may have a known history of polymyalgia rheumatica. Physical examination findings may include fever, tenderness over a nodular temporal artery, decreased pulsation of the artery, and diminished or absent pulses in the upper extremities. Unilateral blindness may occur if untreated. The age of onset is usually older than 50 years of age. An erythrocyte sedimentation rate (ESR) will be greater than 50 mm/hr (Buttaro et al., pp. 1241–1243; Dains et al., p. 404).

30. **(d)** Symptoms of viral conjunctivitis include gradual onset of unilateral (may become bilateral) scratchy sensation in the eye. There is no eye pain, vision changes, or photophobia. Examination of the eye reveals peripheral injection and a watery discharge. Allergic conjunctivitis is bilateral, and the eyes are itchy. There is peripheral injection and a mucoid discharge. There is typically pain and photophobia with corneal abrasion. Subconjunctival hemorrhage is painless and without discharge. There is a splash of blood in the conjunctiva and sclera (Dains et al., pp. 60–61, 63).

31. **(a)** When the woman in an abusive situation is ready to open up, encouragement to discuss the abuse in specific and concrete terms is useful in helping her to validate her experience and to evaluate her level of danger. Asking the woman what she has done differently during the period of time that he has not been abusive implies that she does something to precipitate the abuse. Leaving is often a difficult process for the woman and, until she is ready and has safe plans, may not be the best thing for her to do. Although couple counseling is an option, it is often more beneficial when the abuse has been long term for the woman to seek counseling on her own first (Buttaro et al., pp. 140–141; Hackley et al., pp. 205–209).

32. **(c)** The cycle of violence has three phases: Phase 1 is the tension building state, phase 2 is the acute battering incident, and phase 3 is the honeymoon phase. The honeymoon phase is characterized by the abusive partner acting apologetic and remorseful. He may promise her that the battering will never occur again. When stress or other factors cause conflict and tension, the cycle is repeated (Buttaro et al., p. 138).

33. **(d)** Substance (including alcohol) dependence is defined as a maladaptive pattern of substance use, in the presence of at least three of seven elements, occurring at any time in the same 12-month period. One of these elements of dependence is a persistent desire to use the substance and/or unsuccessful efforts to cut down use. The other answers are elements of substance abuse rather than substance dependence. The person with alcohol dependence may exhibit elements of alcohol abuse (Goldman, p. 174).

34. **(c)** Acanthosis nigricans is a velvety hyperpigmented patch found on the back of the neck, elbows, knuckles, knees, and in the groin and axillary areas in

obese women with moderate to severe insulin resistance. It can, however, also be seen in older adults with malignancies of the gastrointestinal tract and other adenocarcinomas (Buttaro et al., p. 1123; Goldman, p. 1359).

35. **(d)** Interstitial cystitis (IC) or painful bladder syndrome is defined as pelvic pain, pressure, or discomfort, typically associated with persistent urge to void or urinary frequency, in the absence of infection or other pathology. Nocturia is common with IC but incontinence is uncommon. Dyspareunia is frequently seen in women with IC (Association of Reproductive Health Professionals, pp. 5, 8).

36. **(d)** Depression is common in the individual with anorexia nervosa and is seen in about 50% of individuals with bulimia nervosa. Alcohol/drug abuse and a lack of control are characteristic of bulimia nervosa but not anorexia nervosa; intense fear of loss of control predominates in anorexia nervosa. Amenorrhea is one of the diagnostic criteria for anorexia nervosa. Bulimia nervosa may lead to menstrual irregularities but usually not amenorrhea (Buttaro et al., pp. 1399–1340).

37. **(c)** The DSM-IV diagnostic criteria for a Major Depressive Episode include five or more of a group of particular symptoms that present for a 2-week period and represent a change from previous level of function. One of the five symptoms *must* be either depressed mood or loss of interest or pleasure in most activities. The symptoms the woman describes are included in the diagnostic symptoms group as are feelings of worthlessness; excessive guilt, and thoughts about dying or committing suicide (Buttaro et al., p. 1391).

38. **(d)** Selective serotonin reuptake inhibitors such as paroxetine usually have an energizing effect and may lead to insomnia if taken at night. Even when they are taken during the day, they can still cause insomnia. Trazodone is a heterocyclic antidepressant that has a sedative effect, so it is most beneficial to take it at night. These two groups of antidepressants may be used in combination as first line treatment for major depression (Buttaro et al., p. 1394).

39. **(a)** Accident-related injuries kill more children and adolescents than all other causes combined. Almost half of these injury-related deaths are due to motor vehicle accidents. Anticipatory guidance for all individuals in this age group should include advice to always wear seat belts in the car. In addition, adolescents should be counseled to avoid drinking and driving and to avoid riding in a car driven by a person who has been drinking. Of course, counseling in relation to the other answer choices is also important, but they are not related to the leading cause of death for this age group (Ferri, p. 1488; Heron, p. 21).

40. **(b)** ADA recommendations for glycemic, blood pressure, and lipid control to reduce risks for cardiovascular disease in individuals with diabetes mellitus include maintaining HbA1c at less than 7%, blood pressure less than 130/80, LDL cholesterol less than 100 mg/dL, and saturated fat less than 7% of total (ADA, pp. S23, S30).

41. **(c)** In unilateral conductive hearing loss, sound or vibration will lateralize to the impaired ear when conducting the Weber test. This is because room noise will not be as well heard, so detection of vibration in the impaired ear improves. Causes of conductive hearing loss include cerumen impaction, foreign body in ear, otitis media, and perforated eardrum (Bickley, pp. 227, 271).

42. **(b)** Cranial Nerve V Trigeminal has both motor and sensory functions. The motor function is tested by palpating the temporal and masseter muscles while having the patient clench her

teeth. The sensory function is tested by evaluating pain and light touch sensation along the forehead, cheeks, and jaw (Bickley, pp. 674–675).

43. **(b)** Inflammation of the pericardial sac with pericarditis produces a friction rub. This is a high-pitched scratchy sound with two or three short components associated with cardiac movement (Bickley, p. 387).

44. **(d)** Symptoms of pulmonary embolism include sudden onset of shortness of breath, localized pleuritic chest pain, apprehension, bloody sputum production, diaphoresis, fever, and a history of conditions causing risk for emboli. Prolonged immobilization as may occur with long periods of air travel poses a risk. Physical examination findings include restlessness, fever, tachycardia, tachypnea, diminished breath sounds, crackles, wheezing, and pleural friction rub (Dains et al., p. 147).

45. **(c)** Sharp, nonexertional chest pain of short duration is a symptom of mitral valve prolapse. Palpitations and diaphoresis may accompany the pain. Other symptoms may include anxiety and/or panic attacks. The diagnostic hallmark of mitral valve prolapse is a midsystolic click, a late systolic murmur, and an abnormally thickened, redundant mitral valve seen on echocardiogram. Often mitral valve prolapse is asymptomatic. (Buttaro et al., p. 617; Goldman, p. 544).

46. **(c)** An elevated TSH and a suppressed FT_4 are indicative of primary hypothyroidism. Periorbital edema is the only physical examination finding included in the possible answers that is associated with hypothyroidism (Ferri, p. 510).

47. **(b)** The beginning of accelerated growth is usually the first sign of female puberty, but breast budding is the first recognized pubertal change. It is followed by the appearance of pubic hair and axillary hair. Peak growth occurs about 1 year before menarche (Speroff & Fritz, pp. 367–368).

48. **(c)** Viral pharyngitis is characterized by symptoms of malaise, fever, headache, cough, congestion, and fatigue along with sore throat. Physical examination findings include pharyngeal erythema, no or only a small amount of exudate, and negative lymphadenopathy. Bacterial pharyngitis is characterized by sudden onset of severe sore throat and fever. There is usually no cough or congestion. Physical examination findings include fever of 101.5°F or higher, pharyngeal erythema and exudate, and anterior cervical lymphadenopathy. This patient's presentation is typical of viral pharyngitis. She is low risk for group A β-hemolytic streptococcus (GABHS) (Dains et al., pp 28–29).

49. **(b)** Objective information is that detected during physical examination or lab and diagnostic tests. Subjective information includes all aspects of the health history from chief complaint through the review of systems. The problem list may be a combination of objective and subjective information (Bickley, pp. 6, 37–38).

50. **(a)** The presenting signs and symptoms are indicative of hyperthyroidism. Graves' disease comprises 70% of hyperthyroid cases and is seen most commonly in women 20 to 40 years of age. Subacute thyroiditis is a postviral illness that may cause transient hyperthyroidism. The thyroid is usually tender (Buttaro et al., pp. 1170–1172).

51. **(b)** Lipid screening is recommended every 5 years for all adults over 20 years of age. If the screening is a nonfasting total cholesterol and HDL, a follow-up fasting lipid profile should be done in the following situations: total cholesterol 200 mg/dL or more, HDL cholesterol less than 40 mg/dL, test results

borderline in an individual with two or more cardiovascular disease (CVD) risk factors. Risk factors include: female 55 years of age or older, premature menopause, male 45 years of age or older, family history of premature CVD, smoking, hypertension, HDL cholesterol less than 40 mg/dL. CVD risk equivalents include diabetes, stroke or known cerebrovascular disease, peripheral vascular disease, and abdominal aortic aneurysm (Buttaro et al., pp. 1140–1143).

52. **(c)** Presenting symptoms and vital signs are indicative of bacterial pneumonia. Findings of consolidation associated with pneumonia would include increased vocal fremitus, presence of bronchophony, and dullness to percussion over affected lung areas (Dains et al., pp. 146–147).

53. **(d)** The American Cancer Society guidelines recommend colon cancer screening starting at 50 years of age with the option of using a variety of screening techniques. The digital rectal examination and single-specimen fecal occult blood test (FOBT) is not a recommended option for colon cancer screening. The sensitivity of a single sample FOBT is only 5% compared with a sensitivity of 24% with a six-sample home FOBT. Vitamin C may cause false-negative results. Positive results on an FOBT should be followed up with colonoscopy (Bickley, p. 560; Buttaro et al., p. 104).

54. **(b)** The CDC criteria for considering from 5 mm to less than 10 mm induration a positive tuberculin skin test include: HIV infection, recent close contact with a person with active TB infection, fibrotic lesions or evidence of old, healed TB on chest radiograph, or immunosuppression (Buttaro et al., p. 1303).

55. **(d)** Antinuclear antibodies (ANA) may be positive in the individual with an autoimmune disease such as rheumatoid arthritis, systemic lupus erythematosus, scleroderma, or Sjögren's syndrome (Ferri, pp. 876–878, 1441).

56. **(d)** Local and systemic corticosteroids are used in the treatment of systemic lupus erythematosus (SLE). Individuals with SLE should avoid strong sunlight and use sunscreen and protective clothing to avoid extensive exposure that can exacerbate lupus skin rash and active disease. Women with SLE who have unknown or positive antiphospholipid antibodies should not use estrogen-containing contraception. Progestin-only contraceptives, nonhormonal intrauterine contraception, and barrier methods may be acceptable choices. Autoimmune antibody testing is used in the diagnosis of SLE (Buttaro et al., pp. 1254–1257).

57. **(a)** Both the enzyme immunoassay (EIA) and Rapid HIV tests are considered highly sensitive as initial screening tests for HIV infection. Both have the same rate of false positives so must be confirmed by a supplemental test (Western blot or immunofluorescence assay). The Rapid HIV test is FDA approved (CDC, p. 11).

58. **(d)** Hepatitis B surface antibody (HBsAB) appears approximately 4 to 5 months after infection and is an indicator of immunity. HbsAB is also detectable in individuals who have passive immunity secondary to hepatitis B vaccination (Buttaro et al., p. 681).

59. **(b)** The definition for chronic fatigue syndrome includes specific fatigue criteria and four or more symptoms from a set of symptom criteria present for 6 months or more. These symptoms are sore throat, short-term memory or concentration impairment, tender cervical or axillary lymph nodes, headaches of a new type, pattern, or severity, unrefreshing sleep, postexertional malaise lasting more than 24 hours, multijoint pain without swelling or inflammation,

and muscle pain. In addition, the definition includes specific exclusion criteria. There is no evidence of a hormonal relation in chronic fatigue syndrome. The syndrome does occur more commonly in young and middle-aged women (Ferri, p. 209; Houde & Kampfe-Leacher, pp. 30, 35–36).

60. **(b)** A supervised, graded aerobic exercise program has been shown to result in improvements in fatigue and physical functioning in individuals with chronic fatigue syndrome. Cognitive behavioral therapy has also been shown to be of benefit. There is insufficient evidence to support the benefits of antidepressants, corticosteroids, or multivitamins in the treatment of chronic fatigue syndrome (Ferri, p. 209).

◻ REFERENCES

American Diabetes Association. (2009). Standards of medical care in diabetes—2009. *Diabetes Care, 32*(Suppl 1), S14–S61.

Association of Reproductive Health Professionals. (2008). *Screening, treatment, and management of interstitial cystitis/painful bladder syndrome.* Washington, DC: Author.

Bickley, L. (2009). *Bate's guide to physical examination and history taking* (10th ed.). Philadelphia, PA: Lippincott, Williams, & Wilkins.

Buttaro, T., Trybulski, J., Bailey, P., & Sandberg-Cook, J. (2008). *Primary care: A collaborative practice* (3rd ed.). St. Louis, MO: Mosby, Inc.

Centers for Disease Control and Prevention (CDC). (2010). Recommended adult immunization schedule—United States, 2010. *Morbidity and Mortality Weekly Report, 59*(1), 1–4.

Centers for Disease Control and Prevention (CDC). (2006). Sexually transmitted diseases treatment guidelines, 2006. *Morbidity and Mortality Weekly Report, 55*(RR-11), 1–94.

Dains, J., Baumann, L., & Scheibel, P. (2007). *Advanced health assessment and clinical diagnosis in primary care* (3rd ed.). St. Louis, MO: Mosby, Inc.

Ferri, F. (2009). *Ferri's clinical advisor.* St. Louis, MO: Mosby, Inc.

Goldman, L., & Ausiello, D. (2007). *Cecil's textbook of medicine* (23rd ed.). Philadelphia, PA: Saunders.

Hackley, B., Kriebs, J., & Rousseau, M. (2007). *Primary care of women: A guide for midwives and women's health providers.* Sudbury, MA: Jones and Bartlett.

Heron, M. (2010). Deaths: Leading causes for 2006. *National Vital Statistics Reports, 58*(14), 1–100.

Lichtenstein, A., Appel, L., Brands, M. et al. (2006). Diet and lifestyle recommendations revision 2006: A scientific statement from the American Heart Association Nutrition Committee. *Circulation, 114*, 82–96.

Smith, R., Cokkinides, V., & Brawley, O. (2008). Cancer screening in the United States, 2008: A review of current American Cancer Society guidelines and cancer screening issues. *CA: A Cancer Journal for Clinicians, 58*, 161–179.

Speroff, L., & Fritz, M. (2005). *Clinical gynecologic endocrinology and infertility* (7th ed.). Philadelphia, PA: Lippincott, Williams, & Wilkins.

Wynne, A., Woo, T., & Olyaei, A. (2007). *Pharmacotherapeutics for nurse practitioner prescribers* (2nd ed). Philadelphia, PA: F. A. Davis.

2

Gynecology

Beth M. Kelsey

Ann Salomone

Select one best answer to the following questions.

Questions 1 and 2 refer to the following scenario.

A 22-year-old female presents with a complaint of increased vaginal discharge, no itching, and an unpleasant odor. On examination a grayish white discharge is noted at the introitus and adhering to the vaginal walls. There is no erythema.

1. The most likely finding on a wet mount examination will be:

    a. Clue cells
    b. Pseudohyphae
    c. Trichomonads
    d. White blood cells

2. What is the CDC recommended treatment for this client?

    a. Doxycycline
    b. Metronidazole
    c. Ofloxacin
    d. Terconazole

Questions 3 and 4 refer to the following scenario.

A 65-year-old female presents with a complaint of intense itching in her vulvar area for the past month. She has not noticed any abnormal vaginal discharge. On examination, thick white plaques are noted in the vulvar area. There is no discrete mass noted.

3. Initial management for this client should include:

    a. Biopsies of the affected area
    b. Patch testing for allergies
    c. Topical hydrocortisone cream
    d. Vaginal antifungal medication

4. Which of the following is one of the most common causes of vulvar pruritus with a white, wrinkled-appearing lesion involving the entire vulva in a postmenopausal woman?

    a. Lichen sclerorus
    b. Vulvar cancer
    c. Vulvar vestibulitis
    d. Vulvodynia

5. A 20-year-old female presents with a complaint of swelling on one side of her labia. On examination, a 3-cm nontender cystic mass is noted lateral to the posterior vestibule. This is most likely a:

   a. Bartholin's duct cyst
   b. Skene's duct cyst
   c. Hidradenitis suppurativa
   d. *Molluscum contagiosum*

Questions 6 and 7 refer to the following scenario.

A 26-year-old woman and her husband present at the clinic stating that they are having sexual problems. They have been married for 3 months and have not had sexual intercourse. They were reading a book about sexual problems and think that the problem is vaginismus.

6. An examination finding that would confirm that she has vaginismus would include:

   a. Localized tenderness and erythema at the introitus
   b. Involuntary vaginal spasm when a finger is inserted
   c. Presence of a transverse septum in the vagina
   d. Atrophy and friability of the vaginal epithelium

7. Treatment for vaginismus most often includes:

   a. Surgical intervention
   b. Behavioral therapy
   c. Tricyclic antidepressants
   d. Psychotherapy

8. Characteristics of normal vaginal secretions in a reproductive-age woman include:

   a. Adherence to vaginal walls
   b. pH between 5.0 and 6.0
   c. Positive amine whiff test
   d. Presence of lactobacilli

Questions 9 and 10 refer to the following scenario.

A 24-year-old female was seen in the office and treated for her first yeast infection. Symptom relief was achieved. She calls the office 3 months later stating that she thinks she has another yeast infection as her symptoms are exactly the same as before. She states she is in a monogamous relationship with the same sexual partner for the past year.

9. Appropriate management for this woman may include:

   a. Treatment of her and her partner to prevent reinfection
   b. Starting her on a treatment regimen for recurrent yeast infections
   c. Suggesting she try one of the over-the-counter yeast medications
   d. Encouraging her to consider testing for both diabetes and HIV infection

10. Six months later the same woman is seen in the office. She has a positive pregnancy test and another yeast infection. Recommended treatment for a yeast infection during pregnancy is:

    a. Clindamycin vaginal cream one applicator at bedtime for 5 days
    b. Clotrimazole 500 mg vaginal tablet, one tablet in a single application
    c. Fluconazole 150 mg oral tablet, one tablet in a single dose
    d. Terconazole vaginal cream one applicator at bedtime for 7 days

Questions 11 and 12 refer to the following scenario.

A 23-year-old overweight nulliparous female presents with a history of periods every 2 to 3 months for the past 2 years. She has facial acne and is mildly hirsute.

11. The correct term for her menstrual pattern is:

    a. Amenorrhea
    b. Hypomenorrhea
    c. Oligomenorrhea
    d. Metrorrhagia

12. The most likely diagnosis for this client is:

    a. Androgen insensitivity syndrome
    b. Hyperprolactinemia
    c. Polycystic ovarian syndrome
    d. Premature ovarian failure

13. In which of these conditions would you most expect a positive progesterone challenge test?

    a. Androgen insensitivity syndrome
    b. Polycystic ovarian syndrome
    c. Premature ovarian failure
    d. Turner's syndrome

Questions 14 and 15 refer to the following scenario.

A 40-year-old female presents with a complaint of heavy but regular periods occurring at her usual 27 to 28 day intervals. She states that her last period was very heavy and lasted for 8 days. She has had no problems with abdominal pain, menstrual cramping, or pain with sex. She does occasionally feel some pressure in her pelvic area.

14. Expected pelvic examination findings with this client would include:

    a. Diffusely enlarged uterus
    b. Irregularly enlarged uterus
    c. Fixed retroverted uterus
    d. Prolapsed uterus

15. The correct terminology to describe her menstrual pattern is:

    a. Dysfunctional bleeding
    b. Menorrhagia
    c. Metrorrhagia
    d. Polymenorrhea

Questions 16, 17, and 18 refer to the following scenario.

A 32-year-old female presents with a complaint of menstrual cramps that start 1 or 2 days before her period and have gotten worse over the past 6 months. She has had occasional spotting a week before her period and has had increasing pain with sexual intercourse.

16. What is the most likely diagnosis for this client?

    a. Acute salpingitis
    b. Corpus luteum cyst
    c. Endometriosis
    d. Uterine fibroids

17. Expected pelvic examination findings for this client would include:

    a. Diffusely enlarged uterus
    b. Mucopurulent cervicitis
    c. Nodules in the posterior fornix
    d. Stenotic cervical os

18. A definitive diagnostic procedure for the above condition is:

    a. Culdocentesis
    b. Endometrial biopsy
    c. Laparoscopy
    d. Pelvic ultrasound

19. A 10-year-old female has recently developed breast buds. Which of the following statements would be true concerning this young girl?

    a. She is exhibiting signs of precocious puberty
    b. She will most likely start her periods in the next year
    c. She has most likely started her growth spurt
    d. She has probably developed pubic hair

20. Which of the following females, who has never had a period, would be considered to have primary amenorrhea?

    a. A 13-year-old who has no secondary sexual characteristics development

b. A 14-year-old who has develop-
    ment of breast buds but no pubic
    hair
c. A 15-year-old who has beginning
    breast development and some pu-
    bic hair
d. A 16-year-old who has fully devel-
    oped breasts and pubic hair

Questions 21, 22, and 23 refer to the following scenario.

An 18-year-old female, who is not sexually active, has never had a period. She has
normal breast development and both pubic
and axillary hair.

21. Possible causes for her primary amen-
     orrhea include:

     a. Androgen insensitivity syndrome
     b. Asherman's syndrome
     c. Uterine agenesis
     d. Turner's syndrome

22. The genotype for this condition is:

     a. 45 X
     b. 46 XX
     c. 46 XY
     d. 47 XXY

23. A person with this condition would
     have:

     a. Absent or short vagina
     b. Endometrial adhesions
     c. Absent or streak ovaries
     d. Male gonads in the abdomen

Questions 24 and 25 refer to the following scenario.

A 45-year-old female presents with a
6-month history of heavy, irregular periods
every 24 to 30 days and lasting 8 to 10 days.
She is not currently bleeding. Pelvic examination reveals a normal sized, non-tender
uterus and normal adnexa.

24. Which one of the following tests
     would *not* be appropriate in the ini-
     tial evaluation of this problem?

     a. Complete blood count
     b. FSH and LH
     c. Thyroid function test
     d. Transvaginal ultrasound

25. After an appropriate diagnostic evalu-
     ation, this client is determined to have
     dysfunctional uterine bleeding. Ap-
     propriate treatment might include:

     a. Bromocriptine
     b. Conjugated estrogen
     c. Medroxyprogesterone
     d. Prostaglandins

26. A 38-year-old female presents with
     menorrhagia and dysmenorrhea for
     the past 2 years. Physical examination
     reveals a smooth, diffusely enlarged
     uterus that is slightly tender. The most
     likely diagnosis is:

     a. Adenomyosis
     b. Chronic pelvic infection
     c. Endometriosis
     d. Submucosal fibroids

27. Which of the following state-
     ments is true concerning primary
     dysmenorrhea?

     a. Age of onset is usually 5 or more
         years after menarche.
     b. It is often associated with in-
         creased prostaglandin activity.
     c. It is most often associated with
         anovulatory cycles.
     d. Pain often begins 2 to 3 days be-
         fore the period starts.

28. A woman who will be taking a non-
     steroidal anti-inflammatory drug
     (NSAID) for primary dysmenorrhea
     should be told to:

     a. Start the medication several days
         before the expected onset of her
         period
     b. Continue to take the medication
         through the last day of bleeding
     c. Combine two different NSAIDs if
         one is not effective
     d. Avoid these medications if she has
         an aspirin sensitivity

29. A 30-year-old female presents with complaints of monthly premenstrual symptoms that include anxiety, difficulty concentrating, bloating, and breast tenderness. She states that she experiences the same symptoms every month starting about 1 week before her period and resolving soon after her period starts. The most important part of this information in making a diagnosis of premenstrual syndrome is:

    a. Consistency of symptoms
    b. Number of symptoms
    c. Timing of symptoms
    d. Type of symptoms

30. A woman with polycystic ovarian syndrome is at increased risk for:

    a. Cardiovascular disease
    b. Cushing's syndrome
    c. Hyperthyroidism
    d. Ovarian cancer

31. A 52-year-old female with a large uterine fibroid has been placed on leuprolide acetate, a GnRH agonist, to decrease the size of the tumor prior to surgical removal. Which of the following is a common side-effect of this medication?

    a. Breast tenderness
    b. Headaches
    c. Nausea
    d. Hot flashes

32. An 18-year-old female complains of sharp, one-sided, lower abdominal pain that occurs each month and lasts 1 to 2 days. She states that the pain seems to occur about 2 weeks after her period begins each month. A likely cause for this cyclic pain is:

    a. Rupture of the ovarian follicle
    b. Abnormal prostaglandin release
    c. Formation of a corpus luteum cyst
    d. Pelvic congestion syndrome

Questions 33 and 34 refer to the following scenario.

A 32-year-old female presents with no menses for the past 3 months. She has a negative urine pregnancy test, normal TSH, and normal prolactin level. A progesterone challenge test is administered, and she has no withdrawal bleeding. She does have withdrawal bleeding when both estrogen and progesterone are administered.

33. Which of the following laboratory or diagnostic tests is most appropriate as the next step in this client's evaluation?

    a. Cranial imaging—MRI
    b. FSH and LH levels
    c. Hysterosalpingography
    d. Serum estradiol level

34. Potential causes for this client's amenorrhea include:

    a. Androgen insensitivity syndrome
    b. Asherman's syndrome
    c. Hypothalamic dysfunction
    d. Polycystic ovarian syndrome

Questions 35 and 36 refer to the following scenario.

A nonpregnant 27-year-old female presents in your office with complaints of burning with urination and mild suprapubic discomfort for the past 2 days.

35. Which of the following would help you to determine whether she has cystitis or pyelonephritis?

    a. History of recurrent urinary tract infections
    b. Positive nitrites on a urine dipstick
    c. Presence of costovertebral angle tenderness
    d. 10 WBC seen on urine microscopy

36. Laboratory tests and physical examination indicate that she has cystitis. She informs you that this is the fourth episode she has had in the past year and that they always seem to start a day or two after she has sexual intercourse. Options for antibiotic prophylaxis for this patient include all of the following except:

    a. Daily low-dose of nitrofurantoin
    b. One dose of trimethoprim-sulfamethoxazole taken after intercourse
    c. Three day course of trimethoprim-sulfamethoxazole at onset of symptoms
    d. Vaginal estrogen cream one applicatorful three times a week

Questions 37 and 38 refer to the following scenario.

A 52-year-old female presents with a complaint of leaking urine. During questioning she admits that she does notice that it occurs when she laughs or coughs. She has had to give up her aerobics classes because she frequently leaks urine during the exercises.

37. What she is describing best fits the definition for:

    a. Stress incontinence
    b. Overflow incontinence
    c. Urge incontinence
    d. Functional incontinence

38. Treatment options that would be appropriate for the type of incontinence that this client is experiencing include:

    a. Anticholinergic agents
    b. Intermittent catheterization
    c. Limiting fluids during the day
    d. Pelvic floor muscle exercises

39. In which of the following situations is cotesting with cervical cytology plus HPV-DNA testing appropriate?

    a. First time Pap test for 21-year-old female with history of genital warts
    b. Follow-up for 24-year-old female with LSIL Pap test result 6 months ago
    c. Follow-up for 28-year-old female who had LEEP procedure 3 months ago
    d. Screening test for 34-year-old female with no previous abnormal Pap test

40. Appropriate initial management for a 60-year-old female with an atypical squamous cells—cannot exclude high-grade squamous epithelial lesion (ASC-H) Pap test result is:

    a. Colposcopic examination
    b. HPV-DNA testing
    c. Repeat Pap test at 6 and 12 months
    d. Treatment with vaginal estrogen cream and repeat Pap test in 3 months

41. A 25-year-old female has a Pap test result of negative for intraepithelial lesion or malignancy with cellular changes consistent with herpes simplex virus. She states she has never had any symptoms of genital herpes but does get occasional cold sores. Appropriate management would include:

    a. Colposcopic evaluation with biopsy
    b. Culture of cervix to confirm herpes infection
    c. HSV-2 type specific serology
    d. Repeat Pap test in 6 months

42. Which of the following is a major advantage of loop electrosurgical excision procedure (LEEP) over either cryosurgery or laser vaporization for the treatment of preinvasive cervical lesions?

    a. Local anesthesia is rarely needed for the procedure.
    b. There is less risk for postoperative hemorrhage.

c. Excised tissue provides a specimen for further evaluation.

d. There is less risk for postprocedure cervical stenosis.

43. Which of the following is considered a risk factor for cervical cancer?

    a. Smoking one pack of cigarettes per day
    b. Uncircumcised sexual partner
    c. Sexual partner with herpes infection
    d. Use of talcum powder in the genital area

44. Which of the following is *not* considered to be a possible factor in earlier age of menopause?

    a. Autoimmune syndromes
    b. Current smoking
    c. Multiparity
    d. Type I diabetes mellitus

45. A 50-year-old female presents with irregular bleeding at intervals of 20 to 24 days lasting 5 to 6 days and at times heavy over the past 6 months. Her pelvic examination is within normal limits. The endometrium is adequately visualized and is measured to be 7 mm with transvaginal ultrasound. Appropriate management would include:

    a. Insert a levonorgestrel intrauterine system (IUS)
    b. Start on continuous estrogen-progestogen therapy
    c. Start on low-dose combination oral contraception
    d. Refer for further evaluation

46. A 52-year-old female presents with amenorrhea for one year and moderate hot flashes for 6 months. She is interested in bioidentical hormones for relief of her hot flashes and wants to know if they are better for her than other hormones. Appropriate information to provide would include:

    a. Bioidentical hormones do not treat hot flashes as well as conventional hormones.
    b. Bioidentical hormones are safer because they do not increase the risk for breast cancer.
    c. There are no FDA approved bioidentical estrogens currently available.
    d. Topical progesterone cream may not provide adequate protection against endometrial hyperplasia.

47. For the menopausal woman who has a contraindication to estrogen use, a potential alternative treatment for hot flashes that is considered to be safe and effective is:

    a. Bellergal
    b. Fluoxetine
    c. Methyldopa
    d. Raloxifene

48. A 50-year-old healthy, nonsmoking woman on low-dose oral contraceptives asks how she will know when she has reached menopause and does not have to worry about getting pregnant. An appropriate response would be:

    a. She can stay on low-dose oral contraceptives indefinitely as they provide the same hormone dose as menopausal HT.
    b. She can discontinue oral contraceptives now and switch to HT without worrying about pregnancy.
    c. She can continue oral contraceptives until age 55 and then switch to HT if needed.
    d. She should discontinue oral contraceptives for 3 months and then have a test for FSH level.

49. The National Osteoporosis Foundation recommends which of the following for women age 50 and older?

    a. Calcium supplement of 1500 mg in addition to calcium obtained through diet each day
    b. Lower doses of Vitamin D if woman has chronic renal failure

c.   Total of 800 to 1000 IU of Vitamin D every day

d.   Total daily calcium intake of 1800 mg every day

50.   Which of the following does *not* place a woman at increased risk for venous thrombosis?

a.   Bioidentical estrogen
b.   Bisphosphonates
c.   Conjugated estrogen
d.   Estrogen agonists/antagonists (formerly known as SERMs)

51.   A 65-year-old woman currently on cyclic hormone therapy (HT) is at your office for a routine annual examination. She states she has been healthy in the last year and she is having no problems with her HT. On bimanual examination, a 4-cm nontender ovary is palpated. Appropriate management for this woman would include:

a.   Ordering a pelvic ultrasound and referring for further evaluation
b.   Discontinuing HT and repeating the bimanual examination in 2 months
c.   Changing to a continuous HT regimen and rechecking in 2 months
d.   Having her return in 1 year as this is a normal finding for a 65-year-old

52.   Which of the following information would be appropriate to share with a woman concerning risk factors for breast cancer?

a.   Over 50% of women who get breast cancer have a first degree relative who has had breast cancer.
b.   The majority of women who get breast cancer do not have apparent risk factors.
c.   One out of every 12 women in the United States will get breast cancer in her lifetime regardless of family history.
d.   Other risk factors such as early menarche and late menopause are just as important as family history.

53.   As part of instructions on doing breast examination, the nurse practitioner advises the client to inspect her breasts with her hands pressed against her hips. This step is done to:

a.   Check for spontaneous nipple discharge
b.   More easily palpate axillary nodes
c.   Note any muscle weakness in the chest area
d.   Reveal changes in breast contour or symmetry

54.   According to American Cancer Society (ACS) recommendations, women should:

a.   Perform monthly breast self-examination starting in late teenage years
b.   Have clinical breast examination every year beginning at 21 years of age
c.   Begin having annual mammograms at 40 years of age
d.   Consider breast magnetic resonance imaging (MRI) if they have more than one risk factor for breast cancer

55.   For which of the following women would a breast ultrasound be most appropriate?

a.   A 25-year-old with a nontender, palpable mass
b.   A 30-year-old with nipple discharge from one breast
c.   A 40-year-old with breast pain and no palpable mass
d.   A 55-year-old with mammogram showing microcalcifications

Questions 56 and 57 refer to the following scenario.

A 30-year-old female presents with a complaint of a nipple discharge. Her LMP was 2 months ago, and she says it has not been unusual for her to skip periods for 2 to 3 months in the past year. She had a tubal sterilization two years ago after delivering her second child. Her pregnancy test today is negative.

56. If this client's nipple discharge is related to hyperprolactinemia, expected characteristics of the discharge would include its:

    a. Occurring in only one breast
    b. Occurring only with nipple stimulation
    c. Involving multiple ducts
    d. Having a yellow, sticky consistency

57. Additional history that would be pertinent in determining the potential cause for her hyperprolactinemia would include asking about:

    a. Symptoms of hyperthyroidism
    b. Current medications
    c. Symptoms of premature ovarian failure
    d. Family history of diabetes mellitus

58. A 45-year-old female presents with spontaneous bloody nipple discharge from her left breast. On examination, no mass is noted and a bloody discharge is expressed from a single duct. The most likely diagnosis is:

    a. Breast carcinoma
    b. Duct ectasia
    c. Fat necrosis
    d. Intraductal papilloma

59. A 23-year-old female presents with a lump in her breast. On examination, a single, firm, nontender, mobile mass is palpated. The most likely diagnosis is:

    a. Breast carcinoma
    b. Fibroadenoma
    c. Fibrocystic change
    d. Galactocele

Questions 60 and 61 refer to the following scenario.

A 54-year-old woman has been scheduled for a modified radical mastectomy for breast cancer, and has been advised that she will probably be started on tamoxifen after the surgery.

60. In a modified radical mastectomy the:

    a. Breast, axillary nodes, and pectoralis major are removed
    b. Breast and a sampling of lymph nodes are removed
    c. Segment of breast and a sampling of lymph nodes are removed
    d. The tumor and a small amount of surrounding tissue are removed

61. When educating this client concerning the use of tamoxifen, it is important to tell her that:

    a. It should be taken for no more than 6 months after surgery.
    b. Side-effects of this medication include acne and hirsutism.
    c. Use of this medication increases the risk for endometrial cancer.
    d. It cannot be used if cancer cells are estrogen receptor positive.

62. After examining a 25-year-old female who has galactorrhea, you decide to order a prolactin level. All of the following are reasons that this patient should wait until the next morning for the blood test *except*:

    a. It is 3:00 p.m.
    b. You have just finished a thorough breast examination.
    c. She has eaten lunch 3 hours ago.
    d. She took ibuprofen for a headache within the past 24 hours.

63. Which of the following is accurate regarding the use of mifepristone for abortion?

    a. Misoprostol, a prostaglandin, is used with mifepristone to prevent heavy bleeding.
    b. Mifepristone works primarily as an antiprogesterone agent.
    c. Mifepristone is most commonly used for second trimester termination.
    d. Serious adverse reactions to mifepristone have recently been reported.

64. Which of the following aspects of sexual functioning is *least* likely to be affected by the normal changes in a woman's body as she gets older?

a. Amount of lubrication
b. Duration of orgasms
c. Intensity of orgasms
d. Satisfaction with sex life

Questions 65 and 66 refer to the following scenario.

A 30-year-old female presents at the emergency room stating that she was raped earlier that same evening. She appears anxious and smiles nervously while answering questions about the incident. Her breath smells of alcohol and her speech is slightly slurred. She states that her last consensual intercourse was about 1 week ago. She has not used birth control for the past year as she would like to get pregnant.

65. Appropriate documentation by the clinician who performs the sexual assault evaluation would include:

    a. The total number of sexual partners the victim has had
    b. Whether victim's emotional status seems appropriate
    c. The clinician's judgment of whether a rape occurred
    d. Activities of the victim after the rape occurred

66. Which of the following tests would *not* be routinely ordered as part of an assessment of this sexual assault victim?

    a. Serologic test for HIV
    b. Urine pregnancy test
    c. Urine toxicology screen
    d. Pubic hair sampling

67. Translucent nodules on the surface of the cervix are most likely:

    a. Bartholin's gland cysts
    b. Cervical polyps
    c. Epidermoid cysts
    d. Nabothian cysts

68. A 24-year-old female presents in the emergency room with temperature 102°F, blood pressure 80/40 mm Hg, diffuse macular erythema, and desquamation involving her fingers and toes. She has also had vomiting and diarrhea for the past 48 hours. The most likely diagnosis is:

    a. Acute allergic reaction
    b. Acute salpingitis
    c. Toxic shock syndrome
    d. Secondary syphilis

69. Which of the following is an indication for colposcopic examination?

    a. Cellular changes associated with herpes
    b. Cervical leukoplakia
    c. Actinomyces on Pap test if woman has an IUD
    d. Baseline examination for women with HIV

70. Which of the following statements concerning endocervical polyps is true?

    a. The incidence is highest in women younger than 40 years of age.
    b. Intermenstrual bleeding is a common symptom.
    c. Polyps often represent a precancerous condition.
    d. Dyspareunia is a frequent complaint with polyps.

71. Which of the following occurs first in a normal menstrual cycle?

    a. Corpus luteum formation
    b. LH surge
    c. Ovulation
    d. Peak in progesterone level

72. The endometrial phase that corresponds with the luteal ovarian phase is the:

    a. Follicular phase
    b. Menstrual phase
    c. Proliferative phase
    d. Secretory phase

Questions 73 and 74 refer to the following scenario.

A couple has decided to use the fertility awareness method for contraception. They will be combining the use of basal body temperature (BBT), cervical changes, and the calendar method and plan to use abstinence during the woman's fertile days. She has regular periods that occur every 26 to 28 days.

73.   This couple should be instructed to avoid sexual intercourse:

   a.   For 48 hours after a rise of 0.4 degrees in her BBT
   b.   From day 10 through day 20 of each menstrual cycle
   c.   When the woman's cervix feels high in the vagina and soft
   d.   From the end of her period until she has sticky cervical mucus

74.   Other important information for this couple will include that the woman's ovum maintains the potential for fertilization for up to ___ hours, and sperm can survive for up to ___ hours in the female reproductive tract.

   a.   12 ; 24
   b.   24 ; 12
   c.   24 ; 72
   d.   48 ; 96

75.   When fitting a woman for a diaphragm, it is important to remember that when correctly fitted it should:

   a.   Allow a finger tip between it and the pubic arch
   b.   Be small enough to allow for vaginal expansion
   c.   Lie snugly over the pubic arch and under the cervix
   d.   Provide firm tension against the vaginal walls

76.   In making the choice of diaphragm type, the clinician might choose a flat spring diaphragm if the woman has:

   a.   A large pubic arch notch
   b.   Firm vaginal muscle tone
   c.   A retroverted uterus
   d.   A cystocele or rectocele

77.   A woman using a diaphragm for birth control has sexual intercourse at 8:00 p.m. on Friday, 2:00 a.m. on Saturday,

and 8:00 a.m. on Saturday. When can she safely remove her diaphragm for effective contraception, while minimizing problems related to leaving the diaphragm in for extended periods of time?

   a.   10 a.m. on Saturday
   b.   2 p.m. on Saturday
   c.   10 p.m. on Saturday
   d.   8 a.m. on Sunday

Questions 78 and 79 refer to the following scenario.

A 28-year-old female calls your office on Monday morning stating that the condom broke when she and her partner had sexual intercourse Friday afternoon. She is interested in postcoital contraception. She is also interested in starting oral contraception.

78.   In discussing options with this client, it is important to explain that the latest she should wait before initiating hormonal postcoital contraception would be:

   a.   Monday afternoon
   b.   Monday evening
   c.   Tuesday afternoon
   d.   Wednesday afternoon

79.   The woman takes hormonal postcoital contraception Monday afternoon and comes to your office that same day for further information on oral contraception. She states she has had no other unprotected sex since her last period. Information should include that:

   a.   She can start oral contraception on Tuesday and use backup method for 7 days.
   b.   She will need to return in 1 week for a pregnancy test before starting oral contraception.
   c.   She should wait until her next period to start oral contraception.
   d.   She has continued pregnancy protection for at least 1 week after taking hormonal postcoital contraception.

Questions 80 and 81 refer to the following scenario.

A 4-week-postpartum woman who is breastfeeding presents in your office to discuss her contraceptive options. Currently she is breastfeeding on demand and is not providing any supplements. She plans to continue breastfeeding for at least 6 months. She wants to know if she should restart her birth control pills or if she is protected from getting pregnant as long as she is breastfeeding.

80. When counseling this woman concerning the lactational amenorrhea method of contraception, the nurse practitioner should tell her that:

    a. The expected failure rate for this method of contraception is about 20%.
    b. This method is considered effective for only 3 months postpartum.
    c. The woman can rely on this method as long as she is amenorrheic.
    d. Another method should be used if the infant is sleeping through the night.

81. She then asks you if she can restart birth control pills now as she wants to be sure that she does not get pregnant. The best response would be to tell her that:

    a. Combination birth control pills are contraindicated while breastfeeding.
    b. She can start her pills now and use a backup method for 1 month.
    c. She should wait until she has regular periods before restarting her pills.
    d. Progestin-only pills would be a better option than combination pills.

Questions 82 and 83 refer to the following scenario.

An 18-year-old female who wants to start oral contraceptives tells you that she is currently taking oral tetracycline 500 mg bid for treatment of moderate inflammatory acne.

82. She should be advised that:

    a. She should take a 50 mcg estrogen pill while on tetracycline.
    b. She needs to discontinue tetracycline before starting oral contraceptives.
    c. Oral contraceptives may decrease the effectiveness of tetracycline.
    d. Oral contraceptives may also help to improve her acne.

83. The same client returns in 6 months and tells you that the dermatologist has recently started her on isotretinoin as her acne was not improving. She is thinking about quitting her pills in case they are causing her acne. She should be advised that:

    a. She should switch to a barrier method of birth control while on isotretinoin.
    b. Discontinuing pills may cause her to have an exacerbation of acne.
    c. She needs to use a highly effective method of contraception while on isotretinoin.
    d. The effectiveness of her pills may be decreased by the use of isotretinoin.

Questions 84 and 85 refer to the following scenario.

A 22-year-old female has one child and wants to wait 2 to 3 years before having another child. She has been on oral contraceptives for the past 3 years without problems except that she frequently misses pills. She discontinued her pills about 2 months ago and is currently in the third day of her period. She is in the office today for etonogestrel implant (Implanon) insertion.

84. Instructions for this client on use of the etonogestrel implant (Implanon) should include:

    a. It is effective for 5 years.
    b. Most women have regular periods with this method.
    c. She does not need a backup method with her timing of insertion.
    d. This method has the same potential adverse effects as oral contraceptives.

85. Three months later she calls the clinic to say that she is having irregular bleeding and is concerned she might be pregnant. Advice should include:

    a. It is unlikely that the irregular bleeding is caused by the implant, and she probably has an infection.
    b. She should come into the clinic in the next few days for a pregnancy test.
    c. Taking supplemental estrogen for a couple of months may help to stop the irregular bleeding.
    d. Bleeding may indicate that the implant may have migrated and is no longer effective.

86. Which of the following should be performed first when preparing to insert intrauterine contraception (IUC)?

    a. Application of a tenaculum to the cervix
    b. Cleansing of the cervix with antiseptic
    c. A bimanual examination
    d. Sounding of the uterus to determine size

87. Regarding the risk for infection with the insertion of IUC, the clinician would want to keep in mind that:

    a. Insertion during menses has been shown to decrease the incidence of infection.
    b. Prophylactic antibiotics have been shown to significantly decrease the incidence of infection.
    c. The uterine cavity may remain unsterile for several months after IUC insertion.
    d. The greatest risk for pelvic infection associated with use of IUC is within 1 month following insertion.

88. One year after insertion of a Copper T380A IUC, a woman returns to the clinic and is found to be 6 weeks pregnant with the IUC still in place and the string visible. Counseling would include informing her that:

    a. There is a risk the baby will need to be delivered by C-section if the IUC is left in place.
    b. There is an increased risk for preterm labor to occur if the IUC is left in place.
    c. There is an increased risk of congenital anomalies due to the copper in the IUC.
    d. There will be less risk of spontaneous abortion if the IUC is left in place than if removed.

89. A 20-year-old female has been on phenytoin for several years to control her seizure disorder. She has no other problems and needs contraception. Of the following contraceptive methods, the best choice would be:

    a. Combination oral contraceptives
    b. Depot medroxyprogesterone acetate (DMPA) injections
    c. Etonogestrel (Implanon) implants
    d. Progestin-only pills

90. A woman using the contraceptive vaginal ring (NuvaRing) removes the ring during sex in the evening and realizes the next morning that she forgot to reinsert it. If this is week 1 or 2 for this ring she should be advised to:

    a. Discard this ring and insert a new one immediately

b. Discard this ring, wait for withdrawal bleed and insert a new ring
c. Reinsert this ring with no backup needed if it has been out for less than 8 hours
d. Reinsert this ring and use a backup method for 7 days

91. A couple who is considering a vasectomy asks you how soon after the procedure they can discontinue using another form of contraception. The appropriate response would be to say that:

a. Another method of contraception should be continued for 3 to 4 weeks.
b. The procedure is effective immediately so other contraception is not needed.
c. He should have a sperm count about 2 to 3 months after the procedure to see if he is sterile.
d. After 10 ejaculations there will not be any viable sperm in the vas deferens so he will be sterile.

92. A woman has missed three pills in the third week of her pill package. Today is Thursday, and she normally starts her next pack on a Tuesday. In addition to advising this woman to use a backup method for 7 days, she should be instructed to:

a. Finish the current pack and start her new pack as usual
b. Take two pills each day for the next 3 days, then continue pills as usual
c. Continue the current pack until Sunday, then start a new pack
d. Finish the third week of her pack, then start a new pack immediately

93. A 17-year-old female has been on oral contraceptives for 1 year without problems. In the last 2 months she has had some spotting. She has missed no pills and is on no other medications. Initial management should include:

a. Advising her to return if spotting continues in the next cycle
b. Changing her pills to a type with a better endometrial activity
c. Performing a pelvic examination and tests for cervical infections
d. Encouraging her to consider a different method of birth control

94. An advantage of the female condom is:

a. It can be used with a male condom for added protection.
b. It can be used for repeated acts of intercourse.
c. It is made of polyurethane, which is stronger than latex.
d. It is less expensive than most male condoms.

95. A 20-year-old female who is 30% overweight is at the clinic to receive her first DMPA IM injection. Which of the following is true with regard to administering DMPA to this woman?

a. She may need a larger dose than the usual 150 mg.
b. She should return for repeat injections every 2 months.
c. You should massage the injection site well to assure absorption.
d. You should choose a site that assures a deep IM injection.

96. Progestin-only pill users should be instructed:

a. To use a backup method for 48 hours if they are more than 3 hours late taking a pill
b. To throw away the pack and start a new one if two pills are missed in the third week of a pack
c. That ovulation is unlikely to occur with this method if pills are taken at the same time each day
d. That if a period is missed when using progestin-only pills, a pregnancy test should be done

97. A woman who has been receiving DMPA injections for 9 months is 1 week late for her fourth injection.

She states that the last time she had sexual intercourse was 1 week ago. Appropriate management would be:

a. Advising her to use condoms and return at her next menses for an injection
b. Giving the injection and advising her to return if she has no menses in the next month
c. Performing a sensitive pregnancy test and giving the injection if the test is negative
d. Starting her on oral contraceptives and giving the injection when she has her period

98. Which of the following is an appropriate instruction when teaching use of the male condom?

a. Unroll the condom to check for holes before placing it on the penis.
b. Be sure the rolled rim is on the outside when putting the condom on.
c. Do not remove the condom until after the penis loses its erection.
d. Do not use a condom that is more than 1 year past manufacture date.

99. When comparing perfect use failure rates and typical use failure rates, the greatest difference between the two would be seen with which of the following methods?

a. Diaphragm
b. Etonogestrel implant (Implanon)
c. Intrauterine contraception (IUC)
d. Tubal sterilization

100. Noncontraceptive benefits of combination oral contraceptives include a decrease in the risk of:

a. Breast cancer
b. Cervical cancer
c. Colon cancer
d. Ovarian cancer

101. Which of the following demonstrates a normal semen analysis?

a. Sperm concentration 5 million/mL, motility of 60%, and morphology of 40% normal
b. Sperm concentration 15 million/mL, motility of 60%, and morphology of 30% normal
c. Sperm concentration 25 million/mL, motility of 50%, and morphology of 50% normal
d. Sperm concentration 50 million/mL, motility of 40%, and morphology of 40% normal

102. Which of the following statements concerning hysterosalpingography (HSG) is correct?

a. It is usually performed 1 to 2 days after ovulation.
b. It may be therapeutic as well as diagnostic.
c. It involves transabdominal injection of dye into the uterus.
d. It provides for direct visualization of the fallopian tubes.

103. Varicoceles may cause infertility by:

a. Decreasing the sperm count
b. Causing retrograde ejaculation
c. Causing antibody formation
d. Causing erectile dysfunction

104. A 29-year-old female presents for her annual examination. She relates that she and her partner stopped using contraception the previous month and desire to start a family. She has several questions related to fertility awareness and the most optimum time to achieve pregnancy. You advise her that she is most fertile when her cervical mucus is:

a. Clear, watery, and stretchy, at the time it is primarily under the effect of estrogen
b. Clear, watery, and stretchy, at the time it is primarily under the influence of progesterone

c. Opaque, thick, and sticky, at the time it is primarily under the influence of estrogen

d. Opaque, thick and sticky, at the time it is primarily under the influence of progesterone

105. All of the following statements concerning infertility are correct *except*:

a. Cocaine use can impair spermatogenesis.

b. Marijuana use in women can interfere with ovulatory function.

c. Heavy alcohol use in women can decrease fertility.

d. Heavy caffeine use in men may decrease fertility.

106. Clomiphene citrate works as a/an:

a. Dopamine receptor agonist that decreases prolactin levels

b. Estrogen receptor antagonist that enhances gonadotropin secretion

c. Gonadotropin that stimulates ovarian follicular development

d. Gonadotropin releasing hormone that stimulates estradiol secretion

107. A couple presents to you shortly after their marriage. The husband had a vasectomy 3 years ago after the birth of his last child. They are seeking information on the success rate of vasectomy reversals as they would like to have a child together. Which of the following reflects correct information?

a. The success rate for a reversal is directly dependent on the man's current age.

b. Pregnancy rates following vasectomy reversal are generally less than 30%.

c. There is a decreasing chance of reversal success the longer it has been since the vasectomy was done.

d. There is an increased risk of birth defects in pregnancies occurring after a reversal.

108. A common side-effect of clomiphene citrate is:

a. Decreased libido

b. Hirsuitism and acne

c. Hot flashes

d. Weight gain

Questions 109 and 110 refer to the following scenario.

A client presents with complaint of vaginal discharge, dysuria, and postcoital bleeding. Physical examination reveals an erythematous, friable cervix. Urinalysis is within normal limits. Wet mount examination reveals many WBCs.

109. Her male partner has a urethral discharge and a gram stain revealing gram negative diplococcus. Your presumptive diagnosis for your client is:

a. Gonorrhea

b. Trichomoniasis

c. Herpes cervicitis

d. Chlamydia

110. Based on your diagnosis, the CDC recommended treatment for this infection would be:

a. Ceftriaxone 125 mg IM plus azithromycin 1 gram po

b. Metronidazole 2 grams po once

c. Acyclovir 200 mg po five times a day for 7 days

d. Doxycycline 100 mg po bid for 7 days

Questions 111 and 112 refer to the following scenario.

A client presents with several small (1 to 5 mm in size) dome-shaped, waxy papules with umbilicated centers. They are located on her thighs and lower abdomen and do not itch.

111. A likely diagnosis is:

a. Acne vulgaris

b. Erythema nodosum

c.   Folliculitis

d.   *Molluscum contagiosum*

112. Based on the above diagnosis, treatment recommendations include:

a.   Advising the client that the lesions are self-limiting and resolve spontaneously

b.   Applying tretinoin cream to the affected area twice a day for 7 to 14 days

c.   Instructing the client to apply hot soaks and then express the core material

d.   Excision and drainage of the lesions followed by erythromycin for 7 to 14 days

113. Which of the following statements concerning recurrent herpes is true?

a.   A Cesarean section is indicated if a pregnant woman has a recurrence any time after the first trimester.

b.   Systemic symptoms are uncommon during recurrent episodes.

c.   Topical acyclovir is as effective as oral acyclovir for recurrent episodes.

d.   Transmission of the virus is unlikely to occur during the prodromal phase.

114. Which of the following statements about the use of imiquimod 5% cream for the treatment of genital warts is true?

a.   It is the only patient applied therapy for genital warts approved for use in pregnancy.

b.   It is shown to be more effective when combined with cryotherapy.

c.   It should be applied twice a day for 3 days followed by 4 days of no therapy.

d.   The treated area should be washed with soap and water 6 to 10 hours after application.

115. A client who was treated the previous day with benzathine penicillin G for early syphilis calls to report that her muscles ache and she has a fever. Appropriate actions would include:

a.   Advising her to tell all future healthcare providers about this reaction

b.   Consulting a physician about additional tests for possible neurosyphilis

c.   Instructing her to go to the hospital as this may be an allergic reaction

d.   Recommending that she take acetaminophen for relief of her symptoms

116. A 26-year-old client was successfully treated for syphilis one year ago. She has remained abstinent since that time, and you can be fairly certain that she has not become reinfected. Which of the following serologic test results would you expect at this time?

a.   RPR reactive, FTA-ABS negative

b.   RPR nonreactive, FTA-ABS negative

c.   RPR nonreactive, FTA-ABS positive

d.   RPR reactive, FTA-ABS positive

117. A 22-year-old sexually active female presents with complaint of lower abdominal pain since her period ended 2 days ago. She has an intrauterine contraceptive (IUC), had a new sexual partner in the past two months, and does not use condoms. On examination you find that she has cervical motion tenderness. She does not have significant uterine or adnexal tenderness. Appropriate management would include:

a.   Await chlamydia and gonorrhea test results before treating

b.   Discuss referral for evaluation of possible endometriosis

c.   Remove the IUC at this visit and treat for actinomyces

d.   Treat with ceftriaxone 250 mg IM plus doxycycline 100 mg po bid for 14 days

118. An 18-year-old female presents to your STD clinic with a 1-cm, nontender ulcer on her labia minora. She states it began a week ago as a "pimple." A Darkfield examination of exudate

from the ulcerative lesion is positive. Treatment would include:

a. Acyclovir 200 mg five times a day for 7 to 10 days
b. Benzathine penicillin G 2.4 million units IM
c. Cephalexin 250 mg three times a day for 7 to 14 days
d. Triple antibiotic ointment applied three times a day

119. A client presents today for an examination with complaints of dysuria, vaginal discharge, and itching. You obtain a wet mount that demonstrates a pH of 4.0, few WBCs, and pseudohyphae. You would prescribe:

a. Terconazole vaginal cream
b. Metronidazole vaginal gel
c. Clindamycin 2% vaginal cream
d. Metronidazole 2 grams by mouth

120. A 22-year-old female comes to the office because she has noticed "bumps around her vagina." Your examination indicates that these are external genital warts. You would want to explain to her that:

a. Her partner needs a test for subclinical infection.
b. She should have a Pap test every 6 months.
c. There is no therapy that will eliminate the HPV virus.
d. You cannot start treatment until you have her Pap test results.

121. Common presenting symptoms and physical findings with infection caused by *Haemophilus ducreyi* include:

a. A single, painful genital ulcer with inguinal lymphadenopathy
b. Painless ulcerative lesions without regional lymphadenopathy
c. Multiple, nonpruritic condyloma lata in the anogenital area
d. Painful ulcers on mucous membranes and general lymphadenopathy

122. A 28-year-old female presents with the complaint of intense vaginal itching. She complains of a "bad smell" especially after intercourse. Pelvic examination reveals erythema of the vaginal walls and cervix and frothy, yellow-green vaginal discharge. You suspect:

a. Bacterial vaginosis
b. Chlamydia
c. Gonorrhea
d. Trichomoniasis

◻ ANSWERS AND RATIONALES

1. **(a)** The most likely diagnosis for this client is bacterial vaginosis. Characteristics of this infection include an increased, malodorous vaginal discharge. There is usually no itching or erythema. The discharge is typically grayish white, is present at the introitus, and adheres to the vaginal walls. Clue cells are epithelial cells stippled with bacteria that obscure the cell border. This is a classic finding with bacterial vaginosis. Other findings include vaginal pH greater than 4.5, and release of an amine (fishy) odor when KOH 10% is applied to the discharge (CDC, p. 50).

2. **(b)** The CDC recommended treatment for bacterial vaginosis in nonpregnant women is metronidazole 500 mg orally twice daily for 7 days. (CDC, pp. 50–51).

3. **(a)** Several vulvar dystrophies occur more commonly in postmenopausal women. Biopsies are required to evaluate the presence of atypia or malignancy. Vulvar pruritus is one of the common presenting symptoms of vulvar cancer. A mass is common but not always present. Vulvar lesions with cancer may be fleshy, ulcerated, leukoplakic, or warty in appearance (Gibbs et al., pp. 959–960).

4. **(a)** Lichen sclerosus presents with pruritus and a white, wrinkled-appearing lesion that worsens over time, may involve the entire vulva, and may cause adhesions and atrophy of the labia minora. Vulvodynia is a condition presenting with chronic vulvar pain and discomfort. Erythema and "paper cut" erosions may be present. Vulvar vestibulitis syndrome is pain localized to the vulvar vestibule. Localized tenderness and erythema are common. Vulvar cancer may present with intense pruritus and a unifocal plaque, ulcer or mass on the labia majora (NAMS, pp. 52–54, 188).

5. **(a)** The Bartholin's gland ducts are located bilaterally at approximately 5 o'clock and 7 o'clock at the vaginal introitus. These ducts may become obstructed, causing cyst formation. These cysts are usually not tender unless there is infection present (Schuiling & Likis, pp. 417–418).

6. **(b)** Vaginismus is a condition in which there is recurrent or persistent involuntary spasm of the musculature of the outer third of the vagina when a woman either anticipates or experiences attempted entry of the vagina by a penis or other object such as a finger or speculum (Schuiling & Likis, p. 355).

7. **(b)** Psychotherapy and medications are usually not necessary for treatment of vaginismus. Surgical intervention is not indicated. Behavioral therapy is indicated to help the woman learn to voluntarily relax the involved muscles and progressively insert larger objects (one finger, two fingers, etc.), and is usually successful (Gibbs et al., p. 756; Katz et al., p. 188; Schuiling & Likis, p. 357).

8. **(d)** Characteristics of normal vaginal secretions include a pH of 3.8 to 4.2, presence of epithelial cells, lactobacilli, and a variety of aerobic and anaerobic bacteria. Normal vaginal secretions pool in the posterior fornix and do not adhere to the vaginal walls (Schuiling & Likis, p. 405).

9. **(c)** Self-medication with over-the-counter preparations is an acceptable option for women who have been diagnosed previously with a yeast infection and who have a recurrence of the same symptoms. If symptoms persist after using an over-the-counter preparation, or if symptoms recur within 2 months, clinical evaluation is indicated. Treatment of asymptomatic sex partners is not recommended. Because this is only the second yeast infection this woman has had, it would not meet the definition for recurrent yeast infection, which is four or more episodes annually. There is no indication for HIV infection or diabetes testing in this situation (CDC, pp. 54–55).

10. **(d)** Only the topical azoles should be used to treat pregnant women with yeast infections. Many experts recommend 7 days of therapy during pregnancy rather than one of the shorter regimens (CDC, p. 56).

11. **(c)** Oligomenorrhea is infrequent menses at intervals of more than 35 days (Speroff & Fritz, p. 554).

12. **(b)** Polycystic ovarian syndrome (PCOS) is characterized by hyperandrogenism evidenced by hirsuitism and/or hyperandrogenemia, ovarian dysfunction with oligoanovulation and/or polycystic ovaries, and exclusion of related disorders. About 60% of women with PCOS are obese. (Gibbs et al., pp. 689–690; Katz et al., pp. 983–984).

13. **(b)** A positive progesterone challenge test (withdrawal bleed) indicates the presence of endogenous estrogen and an intact endometrium in an individual with amenorrhea. Polycystic ovarian syndrome is the only answer

choice in which both of these are present (Schuiling & Likis, p. 527).

14.   **(b)** Heavier and longer uterine bleeding is the most common symptom with uterine fibroids. The second most common symptom is pelvic pressure. An expected examination finding is an enlarged, irregular, nontender uterus (Schuiling & Likis, pp. 572–573).

15.   **(b)** As described in number 14, the definition of menorrhagia is regular episodes of bleeding that are excessive in amount and duration (Schuiling & Likis, p. 508).

16.   **(c)** Classic symptoms of endometriosis include secondary dysmenorrhea that is progressive, dyspareunia with deep penetration, and infertility. Premenstrual spotting is another common symptom (Schuiling & Likis, p. 580).

17.   **(d)** Signs of endometriosis on pelvic examination include nodularity and tenderness in the posterior fornix along the uterosacral ligaments or on the rectovaginal septum, cervical motion tenderness, and possibly tender enlarged adnexal mass(es). The uterus may be fixed in a retroverted position (Schuiling & Likis, p. 581).

18.   **(c)** Laparoscopy with biopsy of visible endometrial implants is the gold standard for diagnosing endometriosis. Findings can be used to stage the disease (Schuiling & Likis, p. 581).

19.   **(c)** Generally, accelerated growth is the first sign of puberty, followed by breast budding, then appearance of pubic hair, peak growth velocity, and menarche. This sequence of pubertal development generally takes 4.5 years (Speroff & Fritz, pp. 367–368).

20.   **(d)** Primary amenorrhea is defined as no period by age 14 in the absence of secondary sexual characteristics or no period by age 16 regardless of the presence of secondary sexual characteristics (Speroff & Fritz, p. 402).

21.   **(c)** Primary amenorrhea in association with normal breast development and normal pubic and axillary hair growth is often associated with uterine agenesis. This is the second most frequent cause of primary amenorrhea. The individual with androgen insensitivity syndrome will also have primary amenorrhea. Breast development occurs but there is little or no pubic or axillary hair. The female with Turner's syndrome has no secondary sexual characteristic development. Asherman's syndrome is characterized by scarring or adhesions in the intrauterine cavity. This is usually the result of uterine surgical procedures or pelvic infection. This would be an unlikely cause for an 18-year-old who has never had a period and is not sexually active (Katz et al., pp. 933, 937–942; Speroff & Fritz, pp. 419–423).

22.   **(b)** The individual with uterine agenesis has a normal female karyotype of 46XX. The individual with androgen insensitivity syndrome has a male karyotype of 46XY. 45X is seen with Turner's syndrome. 47XXY is seen with Klinefelter's syndrome in males (Katz et al., pp. 933, 938–940; Speroff & Fritz, pp. 421–424).

23.   **(a)** The individual with complete uterine agenesis will have a shortened or absent vagina. She will have normal ovaries. Endometrial adhesions are seen with Asherman's syndrome. The individual with Turner's syndrome will have absent or streak ovaries. The individual with Androgen insensitivity syndrome will have male gonads in the abdomen (Katz et al., pp. 938–942; Speroff & Fritz, pp. 419–424).

24.   **(b)** The complete blood count with differential and platelet count can determine if anemia is present. Also, abnormalities may indicate the need for

further evaluation for possible blood dyscrasias or thrombocytopenia. Thyroid function tests may reveal hypothyroidism, which is one of the more common systemic causes for abnormal uterine bleeding. Transvaginal ultrasound and sonohysterogram may be ordered to evaluate the uterine cavity for endometrial polyps, submucous leiomyomas, and other lesions (Katz et al., pp. 919–920; Speroff & Fritz, pp. 555–556).

25. **(c)** Treatment options for chronic dysfunctional uterine bleeding include low-dose oral contraceptives, medroxyprogesterone acetate, prostaglandin synthetase inhibitors, D&C, endometrial ablation, and hysterectomy. Conjugated estrogen may be administered intravenously or orally for treatment of acute dysfunctional bleeding (Schuiling & Likis, pp. 520–525; Speroff & Fritz, pp. 557–560).

26. **(a)** Adenomyosis is the growth of endometrial tissue in the myometrium. Dysmenorrhea may begin up to 1 week before menses and persist until after the period is over. Heavy bleeding is also associated with adenomyosis. Pelvic examination often reveals a diffusely enlarged, smooth uterus that is tender especially at the time of menses (Katz et al., p. 449; Schuiling & Likis, pp. 577–578).

27. **(b)** Primary dysmenorrhea is menstrual pain without related pathology. The cause of primary dysmenorrhea is increased prostaglandin production in the endometrium. Onset is usually within 1 to 2 years of menarche when ovulatory cycles are established. Pain usually begins with onset of menstrual flow and may last up to 48 hours, when most prostaglandin is released (Lowdermilk & Perry, p. 147; Speroff & Fritz, p. 540).

28. **(d)** Studies have shown that beginning NSAIDs at the start of menses is as effective as starting before menses starts. Most women only need medication for the first 2–3 days of bleeding when prostaglandin release would be the highest. Changes in dosage or type of NSAID may be considered if the first one is not effective. Women with hypersensitivity to aspirin should not take NSAIDs (Katz et al., p. 903; Speroff & Fritz, p. 540).

29. **(c)** The diagnosis of PMS can be made when symptoms consistent with PMS occur in the luteal phase, resolve shortly after menses onset, are absent during the follicular phase, and reoccur in the luteal phase. The symptoms must have a negative impact on some aspect of the woman's life and other diagnoses that might better explain the symptoms should be excluded (Lowdermilk & Perry, pp. 151–152; Speroff & Fritz, pp. 531–532).

30. **(a)** Epidemiologic studies have demonstrated an increase in cardiovascular disease and diabetes in older women previously diagnosed with chronic anovulation and polycystic ovarian syndrome (Speroff & Fritz, pp. 484–485; Schuiling & Likis, p. 534).

31. **(d)** GnRH agonists such as leuprolide acetate act by causing a hypoestrogenic state in the woman. This drug may be used prior to surgery to provide temporary relief from bleeding and to decrease the size of the uterine fibroid. Because side-effects include those seen with estrogen deficiency, including hot flashes and bone mineral depletion, this drug is only recommended for short-term therapy (Katz et al., p. 446; Speroff & Fritz, p. 564).

32. **(a)** Midcycle pelvic pain is often associated with rupture of the ovarian follicle at the time of ovulation. This is called mittelschmerz (Schuiling & Likis, p. 474).

33. **(b)** The absence of a withdrawal bleed after a progesterone challenge, but occurrence of bleeding after estrogen and progesterone are administered, suggests that the woman has inadequate endogenous estrogen production but an intact endometrium and outflow tract. Hypoestrogenism may result from problems anywhere in the hypothalamic-pituitary-ovarian axis. Elevated FSH and LH indicate that the problem is ovarian. Normal or low FSH and LH indicate that the problem is either in the hypothalamus or pituitary gland. An estradiol level is not necessary as hypoestrogenism has already been established, and a hysterosalpingography is not needed as an intact endometrium and outflow tract have been established (Speroff & Fritz, pp. 404–417).

34. **(c)** Hypothalamic dysfunction results in differing levels of hypoestrogenism depending on the severity of the dysfunction. Hypothalamic dysfunction may be caused by chronic disease, anorexia nervosa, stress, excessive exercise, malnutrition, or rarely, an anatomic lesion. The individual with androgen insensitivity syndrome would have primary amenorrhea. Although she may have some withdrawal bleeding with Asherman's syndrome, the fact that she has had no menses, or even spotting for 3 months, makes this less likely. The individual with polycystic ovarian syndrome, will have a withdrawal bleed with a progesterone challenge unless there is significant hyperandrogenemia causing endometrial decidualization (Katz et al., pp. 942–945, 949; Speroff & Fritz, pp. 404–417).

35. **(c)** Costovertebral tenderness is usually present with pyelonephritis. It would not be present with cystitis (Buttaro et al., p. 752).

36. **(d)** Recurrent cystitis may be managed with a variety of prophylactic regimens using antibiotics known to be effective in treating urinary tract infections. These regimens include a low-dose (subtherapeutic) antibiotic taken daily or three times each week, antibiotic taken after sexual intercourse if UTI precipitated by sex, and patient-initiated antibiotics for 3 days starting at the onset of symptoms. Topical estrogen may be beneficial for postmenopausal women with signs and symptoms of vulvovaginal atrophy (Buttaro et al., p. 757)

37. **(a)** Stress incontinence is the involuntary loss of urine during activities that increase intra-abdominal pressure such as laughing, coughing, and jumping. Urge incontinence is involuntary loss of urine associated with a sudden, strong urge to void. Overflow incontinence is a result of urinary retention with bladder distention and overflow of urine. Functional incontinence results from medically reversible causes such as delirium, infection, medications, and restricted mobility (Buttaro et al., p. 745).

38. **(d)** Nonsurgical treatment for stress incontinence usually involves efforts to enhance the ability of the pelvic floor muscles to compensate for increased intra-abdominal pressure. These include muscle strengthening exercises, improving estrogen status, electrical stimulation of the muscles, and use of alpha-adrenergic agonists. Bladder retraining and anticholinergic-antimuscarinics are used in treatment of urge incontinence. Intermittent catheterization may be used with bladder retention (Buttaro et al., pp. 747–749).

39. **(d)** Cotesting with a combination of cervical cytology plus HPV-DNA testing is appropriate for women 30 years of age and older. Cotesting is not recommended for women younger than 30 year of age because of the high prevalence of HPV infections

in sexually active women in this age group. Women 30 and older with both a negative cytology and negative HPV DNA test should be rescreened no sooner than 3 years (ACOG, 2009, p. 7).

40. **(a)** Colposcopic evaluation is recommended for all women who have an ASC-H Pap test result (ACOG, 2008, pp. 1469–1470).

41. **(c)** The Pap test is not a very sensitive test for herpes simplex but it is a very specific indicator when present. Infection can be confirmed with a positive HSV-2 type specific serology. This patient's test for HSV-1 antibodies will likely also be positive because she has history of cold sores. Colposcopy is not indicated nor is a repeat Pap test sooner than routine. Because of the intermittent nature of herpes viral shedding a culture is not recommended (Hatcher et al., p. 574).

42. **(c)** A major advantage of LEEP is that it is not a destructive technique, so the excised tissue is suitable for further histologic examination. Both cryosurgery and laser vaporization destroy the transformation zone so a specimen is not available for further diagnostic evaluation (Katz et al., pp. 753–754; Gibbs et al., p. 999).

43. **(a)** Several studies have demonstrated an increased risk of cervical cancer among smokers. Potential mechanisms of connection between smoking and cervical cancer include nicotine and cotinine having a direct effect on cervical mucus, the oncogenicity of HPV being enhanced by tobacco smoke, and smoking causing local immunosuppression within the cervix. The other three choices have not been shown to increase the risk for cervical cancer (Gibbs et al., pp. 971–972).

44. **(c)** Some genetic variations, environmental exposures, medical conditions, and lifestyle factors may contribute to the earlier occurrence of menopause. These include, but are not limited to: current smoking, autoimmune syndromes, cancer therapies, type 1 diabetes mellitus, epilepsy, adverse socioeconomic conditions, and nulliparity (NAMS, p. 19).

45. **(d)** The perimenopausal woman having abnormal uterine bleeding needs endometrial evaluation. The initial evaluation may include endometrial biopsy and/or transvaginal ultrasound. Endometrial thickness greater than 5 mm or suboptimal visualization of the uterus requires further evaluation. This may include saline infusion sonohysterogram or hysteroscopy (Gibbs et al., pp. 665–668; NAMS, pp. 32–33).

46. **(d)** Bioidentical hormones may offer the same relief for hot flashes as conventional hormones but no studies have shown they are safer to use. 17β estradiol is available in some FDA approved formulations. Studies have demonstrated that while progesterone creams can be absorbed through the skin, serum levels are not high enough to protect against endometrial hyperplasia if also taking estrogen (NAMS, pp. 217–218, 225).

47. **(b)** Several nonhormonal prescription medications may be effective for hot flashes in women who cannot take estrogen. These include selective serotonin reuptake inhibitors (SSRIs) such as fluoxetine; serotonin-norepinephrine reuptake inhibitors (SNRIs) such as venlaxafine; gabapentin, and clonidine. NAMS recommends against the use of Bellargal or methyldopa because of limited efficacy data and potential adverse effects. Raloxifine is an estrogen agonist/antagonist (formerly known as a SERM) with a

common side-effect of hot flashes (NAMS, pp. 39–40).

48. **(c)** Approximately 50% of nonsmoking women will reach menopause by age 51. About 90% reach menopause by age 55. Healthy women who do not smoke can stay on low-dose oral contraceptives until age 55 and may benefit from reduction of vasomotor symptoms, irregular bleeding, as well as decreased risk for endometrial cancer. After age 55 if menopausal symptoms warrant it she can be switched to HT (NAMS, p. 205; Hatcher et al., p. 706).

49. **(c)** The National Osteoporosis Foundation (NOF) recommends that women older than 50 years of age consume at least 1200 mg of elemental calcium daily through diet and supplements. Calcium intake of greater than 1200–1500 mg each day shows no significant additional benefit for bones and may increase the risk for development of kidney stones or cardiovascular disease. NOF recommends daily intake of 800 to 1000 IU of vitamin D for adults age 50 and older. Adults with malabsorption conditions such as celiac disease or with renal insufficiency may require higher doses of vitamin D (NOF, p. 17).

50. **(b)** Estrogen agonists/antagonists (formerly known as SERMS) such as raloxifine increase the risk for deep vein thrombosis to the same extent as estrogens. There is no evidence that bioidentical estrogen is any safer in relation to adverse effects than other estrogen formulations. Bisphosphonates such as alendronate do not increase the risk for deep vein thrombosis (NAMS, pp. 125, 218).

51. **(a)** Ovaries are approximately 3 cm long, 2 cm wide, and 1 cm thick in the adult woman during the reproductive years. After menopause the ovaries decrease in size to approximately 1 to 2 cm. It is recommended that the postmenopausal woman with a palpable ovary be further evaluated (Katz et al., p. 55; Seidel et al., p. 581).

52. **(b)** Risk factors identify only 15 to 25% of women who will eventually develop breast cancer. The majority of women who get breast cancer do not have apparent risk factors except for gender and age. Only 5 to 10% of breast cancer is familial. Early menarche and late menopause are less significant as risk factors than family history. One in eight women in the United States will develop breast cancer in her lifetime (Gibbs et al., pp. 932, 935; Speroff & Fritz, p. 591).

53. **(d)** Hands are pressed on hips during inspection of the breasts to emphasize any changes in the shape or contour of the breasts (Katz et al., p. 39; Seidel et al., p. 498).

54. **(c)** The American Cancer Society recommends that women begin annual mammography at age 40. Women should be told about the benefits and limitations of breast self-examination starting in their early 20s, but it is acceptable to not do breast self-examination or to perform it irregularly. Clinical breast examination is recommended during routine periodic examinations every 2 to 3 years in women in their 20s and 30s and annually for women 40 years of age or older. Mammograms with MRI may be considered for annual screening in women who have a known or estimated high-risk mutation status or a history of high-dose radiation at a young age (Smith et al., pp. 101–103).

55. **(a)** The main function of breast ultrasound is to differentiate between a solid and cystic mass. It may also be useful in the differential diagnosis of masses in the dense breast tissue of younger women (Gibbs et al., p. 939).

56. **(c)** The nipple discharge caused by hyperprolactinemia usually occurs in both breasts, involves multiple ducts, is spontaneous, and is milky and thin in consistency (Schuiling & Likis, 326; Lowdermilk & Perry, pp. 256–257).

57. **(b)** Several medications can cause an increase in prolactin release with resultant galactorrhea. These include but are not limited to tricyclic antidepressants, phenothiazine, metoclopramide, amphetamines, opiates, combination oral contraceptives, and several antihypertensives (Speroff & Fritz, p. 583).

58. **(d)** The most common cause of spontaneous serous or bloody nipple discharge from a single duct is an intraductal papilloma. Of course, a malignancy must always be considered. The discharge associated with duct ectasia is most often multicolored and sticky. There is no nipple discharge associated with fat necrosis or fibroadenomas (Gibbs et al., pp. 942–944).

59. **(b)** Fibroadenomas are the second most common benign tumor of the breast. They are the most common benign breast tumor in adolescents and women in their 20s. They are usually single and are firm or rubbery, nontender, and mobile. They do not change in size with the menstrual cycle. Fibrocystic changes are the most common of the benign breast conditions. Symptoms of fibrocystic changes include breast tenderness that is cyclical and often bilateral. Nodularity is a common physical finding. This condition is most common between the ages of 20 and 50. A galactocele is a discrete, milk filled, cystic or firm mass in the breast of a lactating or recently lactating woman (Gibbs et al., pp. 942–943; Schuiling & Likis, pp. 322, 328–330).

60. **(b)** A modified radical mastectomy is the removal of the entire breast

and a sample of lymph nodes, sparing the pectoral muscles. Choice "a" describes a radical mastectomy. Choice "c" describes a partial mastectomy. Choice "d" describes a lumpectomy. The modified radical mastectomy and lumpectomy are the two most common surgical approaches for the treatment of breast cancer (Lowdermilk & Perry, pp. 264–265).

61. **(c)** The use of tamoxifen does increase a woman's risk for endometrial cancer and deep vein thrombosis. Tamoxifen is an estrogen agonist/antagonist used as adjuvant therapy after surgery for postmenopausal women with breast cancers that have estrogen-positive receptors. Women should continue the medication for at least 5 years. Side-effects include hot flashes, nausea and vomiting, fluid retention, weight gain, and thrombocytopenia (Lowdermilk & Perry, p. 267).

62. **(d)** Breast stimulation, exercise, and stress can cause a surge in prolactin level. It is recommended that the blood sample be drawn in the morning. The patient should fast for 12 hours prior to having blood drawn. Several medications can impact the prolactin level. Ibuprofen is not considered to be one of them (Chernecky & Berger, pp. 906–907).

63. **(b)** Mifepristone acts as an antagonist to block the effect of progesterone. It is 95% effective when used in combination with the prostaglandin misoprostol in the first 9 weeks of pregnancy. It is not currently FDA approved for second trimester abortion. Misoprostol works by causing uterine contractions to help expel the uterine contents. No serious adverse reactions have been reported with the use of mifepristone (Hatcher et al., pp. 645–648).

64. **(d)** The physical changes of aging may have an impact on a woman's

sexuality in the following ways: vaginal lubrication may become less in volume; stimulation may take a longer period of time to occur; orgasms may be shorter; and orgasmic contractions may decrease in strength. A woman's satisfaction with her sex life seems to be most affected by her feelings for her partner, whether her partner has sexual problems, and her overall sense of well-being. Some women have an increased sexual interest with age (Association of Reproductive Health Professionals, pp. 8–10).

65. **(d)** It is important to obtain and document information concerning activities after the sexual assault such as bathing, changing clothes, and using mouthwash, as these activities may affect the presence of evidence. The total number of partners the victim has ever had is irrelevant to treatment or the collection of evidence, and may be used against the woman if she goes to trial. Questions about more recent sexual activity are appropriate. It is not unusual for emotional status to change quickly from crying to being calm and controlled. Emotional status should be assessed, but judgments as to appropriateness of emotional behavior should not be included in documentation. Rape and sexual assault are legal terms that should not be used in medical documentation unless quoting the victim. (Lowdermilk & Perry, pp. 139–142; US Department of Justice Office on Violence Against Women, pp. 28–29, 83).

66. **(c)** Urine or blood toxicology screening for drugs/alcohol is generally not advised as part of the sexual assault assessment unless necessary in providing care for the woman. This information may be used against the victim if she goes to trial. Baseline testing for STDs (including HIV), and for pregnancy if no contraception is being used, are usually performed as part of sexual assault assessment. Of course, none of these tests should be performed without the woman's informed consent (Lowdermilk & Perry, pp. 140–142; US Department of Justice Office on Violence Against Women, pp.101–102, 105–111).

67. **(d)** Nabothian cysts are small translucent yellow or white nodules on the surface of the cervix. These are retention cysts of the endocervical glands and are a normal variation (Schuiling & Likis, p. 119).

68. **(c)** Toxic shock syndrome (TSS) is caused by absorption of toxins produced by colonized *Staphylococcus aureus*. It is rare but may be fatal and occurs most frequently in menstruating women. Clinical presentation includes fever of 102°F or greater, hypotension, diffuse macular erythema resembling a sunburn, and desquamation of the skin on fingers, toes, palms and soles. Vomiting and diarrhea are often present at the onset of illness. Other signs and symptoms may include severe myalgia, headache, sore throat, and disorientation (Gibbs et al., pp. 611–612).

69. **(a)** Colposcopic examination is recommended in some situations even if the Pap test is normal. These situations include the presence of cervical leukoplakia (white lesions visible to the naked eye) and persistent or unexplained cervical bleeding. Women infected with HIV should have a Pap test twice in the first year after diagnosis and then annually. A baseline colposcopy is not recommended. Colposcopic evaluation is not indicated for a woman with changes suggestive of herpes or actinomyces and an otherwise normal Pap test (ACOG, p. 5; Hatcher et al., p. 574).

70. **(b)** Intermenstrual bleeding and postcoital spotting are often the presenting symptoms of endocervical polyps. These polyps occur most frequently

in multiparous women older than 40 years of age. The majority of polyps are benign. Dyspareunia is not a common presenting symptom (Lowdermilk & Perry, p. 282; Schuiling & Likis, p. 571).

71. **(b)** The order of the events in a normal menstrual cycle would be LH surge, ovulation, corpus luteum formation, and peak in progesterone level (Lowdermilk & Perry, p. 96).

72. **(d)** The endometrial phases in the menstrual cycle include the proliferative phase corresponding with the follicular ovarian phase, the secretory phase corresponding with the luteal ovarian phase and the menstrual phase (Lowdermilk & Perry, p. 96).

73. **(c)** Near ovulation the cervix feels higher or deeper in the vagina and is soft, open, and wet. BBT should remain elevated at least 0.4°F above the baseline for 3 days to mark the end of the fertile period. When using the calendar method, the first day of fertility is calculated by subtracting 18 days from the length of the shortest cycle, and the last day of fertility is calculated by subtracting 11 days from the longest cycle. For this couple that would be days 8 through 17 of each menstrual cycle. Before ovulation, the only days that are considered safe are the dry days after menses. The couple should not have unprotected intercourse once they note onset of sticky mucus until the evening of the fourth day after peak mucus day. Peak mucus day is the last day of the clear, slippery spinnbarkeit type mucus (Lowdermilk & Perry, pp. 210–212).

74. **(c)** The ovum maintains the potential for fertilization for up to 24 hours. Sperm may remain viable in the female reproductive tract for up to 72 hours (Speroff & Fritz, pp. 236, 241).

75. **(a)** An appropriately sized diaphragm should not be too tightly pressed against the pubic arch, but allow for one finger tip to fit between the inside of the pubic arch and the anterior edge of the diaphragm. The largest size that is comfortable should be used as vaginal depth increases during sexual arousal and a too small diaphragm may not stay in place. The diaphragm should fit snugly but without tension against the vaginal walls (Hatcher et al., p. 330).

76. **(b)** The flat spring diaphragm has gentle spring strength and is suitable for the woman who has firm vaginal muscle tone. It may also provide a better fit for the woman who has a shallow notch behind the pubic bone. An arcing spring diaphragm may provide a better fit for the woman with a cystocele, rectocele, or retroverted uterus (Hatcher et al., p. 320).

77. **(b)** The diaphragm should be left in place for at least 6 hours after the last sexual intercourse as sperm can survive for a few hours in the vagina. The diaphragm should not be left in place longer than 24 hours because of the potential risk for TSS. She should, of course, have used an additional applicator full of spermicide in the vagina before the second and third time she had sexual intercourse (Hatcher et al., p. 319).

78. **(d)** For the maximum effectiveness, hormonal postcoital contraception pills should be taken as soon after unprotected sexual intercourse as possible. Studies indicate that it is an effective option up to 120 hours after unprotected sex (Hatcher et al., p. 104).

79. **(a)** Hormonal postcoital contraception provides no protection against pregnancy in the days or weeks after treatment. Women who want to start

oral contraception can take the first pill the day after postcoital contraception is used and use a backup method for the first 7 days of pills (Hatcher et al., p. 106).

80. **(d)** The lactational amenorrhea method has a 1 to 2% failure rate as contraception, for up to 6 months postpartum, in the breastfeeding woman who is amenorrheic and who is not supplementing feedings. To be effective, the infant must be fed on demand without bottle-feeding supplements and only minimal cup or spoon-feeding supplements. Another method of contraception should be initiated when the woman resumes menstruation, decreases breastfeeding (e.g., baby sleeping through the night), begins any bottle-feeding, or when the baby turns 6 months old (Hatcher et al., pp. 407–409).

81. **(d)** Progestin-only pills have been shown to have no adverse effect on lactation even when started in the first week postpartum. However, the general recommendation is to wait until 6 weeks postpartum. While breastfeeding is not an absolute contraindication to the use of combination oral contraceptives, their use has been shown to decrease milk supply and may alter the composition of breast milk. If she plans to use combination oral contraceptives with the resumption of menses, they should be started with the first postpartum period as ovulation may occur even when periods are irregular (Hatcher et al., pp. 416–418).

82. **(d)** There is no evidence that broad spectrum antibiotics such as tetracycline decrease the effectiveness of oral contraceptives. Long-term use of tetracycline for acne treatment while taking oral contraceptives does not necessitate a higher oral contraceptive dose or the use of a backup method. Oral contraceptives do not decrease the effectiveness of tetracycline. Oral contraceptives may help with improvement of acne (Hatcher et al., pp. 205, 237).

83. **(c)** Oral contraceptives tend to improve acne by suppressing endogenous androgen production. This effect comes from a decrease in free testosterone and increase in sex hormone binding globulin levels. Therefore it is unlikely that the client's pill use is causing her acne. There is also no indication that discontinuing her pills while on isotretinoin would result in an exacerbation of her acne. Isotretinoin is a known teratogen. Use in pregnancy has resulted in the birth of infants with severe neurologic defects. Oral contraceptives or one of the other highly reliable contraceptive methods should be used while taking isotretinoin. Some clinicians recommend an additional backup method to assure prevention of pregnancy (Wynne et al., pp. 590–591).

84. **(c)** The etonogestrel implant (Implanon) is effective for 3 years. If inserted in days 1 through 5 of the menstrual cycle, a backup method is not required. This is a progestin-only method, so it can be used by women who have contraindications to or cannot tolerate estrogen-containing methods. Irregular bleeding is common with this method (Hatcher et al., pp. 152–154).

85. **(c)** Irregular bleeding is common with etonogestrel implants, especially in the first few months. Unless other symptoms cause concern, there is no need for a pregnancy test or tests for infections. Supplemental estrogen or prostaglandin inhibitors may be useful in treating the irregular bleeding (Hatcher et al., p. 154).

86. **(c)** It is important to perform a careful bimanual examination prior to IUC insertion. Undetected posterior

uterine position is the most common reason for perforation at the time of insertion. The other answer choices would then be performed in the following order; clean the cervix with antiseptic, apply a tenaculum, and sound the uterus (Hatcher et al., p. 132).

87. **(d)** The risk of pelvic infection related to IUC is limited to the first 20 days after insertion. Risk for infection related to the IUC after this time period is low. Data do not indicate any benefit to using prophylactic antibiotics at the time of insertion. The IUC may be inserted at any time in the menstrual cycle if there is reasonable assurance that the woman is not pregnant. There is no impact on infection risk related to when in the cycle the IUC is inserted. The uterine cavity is sterile again in a short period of time after IUC insertion (Hatcher et al., pp. 125–126, 131).

88. **(b)** There is an increased risk for preterm labor to occur if the IUC is left in place during pregnancy. There is not an indication for C-section delivery and no risk for congenital anomalies related to the copper in the IUC. IUC removal, when the string is visible, is not associated with an increased risk of spontaneous abortion. There is an increased risk of spontaneous abortion if the IUC is not removed (possibly a septic abortion) or if removal is attempted when the string has drawn up into the uterus (Hatcher et al., p. 125; Katz et al., pp. 312–313).

89. **(b)** Depot medroxyprogesterone acetate (DMPA) effectiveness is not decreased by the concomitant use of phenytoin or other antiseizure medications. DMPA has been shown to decrease seizure activity probably due to the sedative properties of progestin. Most of the antiseizure medications (except sodium valproate) are liver enzyme inducers that cause breakdown of estrogen or progestin. These medications can significantly decrease the effectiveness of etonogestrel implants, combination oral contraceptives, and progestin-only pills (Hatcher et al., pp. 151, 160, 186, 235–237).

90. **(d)** The same ring can be reinserted and a backup method should be used for 7 days. She may want to consider emergency contraception. Also discuss with her that the ring does not need to be removed during sex as most women and partners do not have discomfort due to the ring being in the vagina during sexual intercourse. If it is removed, it should be reinserted within 3 hours (Hatcher et al., pp. 289–290).

91. **(c)** Sperm may not be cleared from the vas deferens after vasectomy for 2 to 3 months or up to 20 ejaculations. A sperm count should be done after this time period or number of ejaculations to assure that no viable sperm remain in the vas deferens (Hatcher et al., p. 392).

92. **(d)** If a woman misses two or more pills (especially those with less than 30 mcg estrogen) in the third week of her pill pack she should finish the rest of the hormonal pills in her pack. She should not take the usual 7 days off of hormonal pills but should start a new pack as soon as she finishes that third week of her current pack. In addition, she should use a backup method until she has taken seven consecutive pills (Hatcher et al., p. 252).

93. **(c)** The fact that this teenager has been taking oral contraceptives for 1 year without spotting, and now is having a problem, should alert the clinician that something other than pills may be the cause. Especially with teenagers, the possibility of chlamydia should be considered (Hatcher et al., p. 242).

94. **(c)** The female condom is made of polyurethane, which is stronger than latex. It is intended for one-time use. Use along with a male condom is not recommended as friction between the two condoms increases risk for displacement or breakage of the male condom. Female condoms are more expensive than male latex condoms (Hatcher et al., p. 318).

95. **(d)** Depot medroxyprogesterone acetate (DMPA) IM formula should always be injected deeply into the deltoid or gluteus maximus muscle to assure optimal effectiveness. In an obese client, the deltoid muscle might be better than the gluteal muscle to assure that administration is deep IM. Massaging the area after injection may lower effectiveness. The dosage is 150 mg and the timing is every 3 months regardless of a woman's weight (Hatcher et al., p. 168).

96. **(a)** Ovulation is not always suppressed with progestin-only pills even when they are taken at the same time each day. One of the other main mechanisms of action of progestin-only pills is thickening and decreasing the amount of cervical mucus, making sperm penetration more difficult. This mechanism of action requires that pills be taken very regularly. Cervical mucus may not maintain this quality if pills are taken as little as 3 hours late, but will return within 48 hours of taking the late pill (Hatcher et al., pp. 182, 188).

97. **(c)** Ovulation is suppressed for at least 14 weeks after a DMPA injection. If the interval between injections is greater than 14 weeks the clinician should determine that the client is not pregnant before administering the next injection. If the last unprotected sex was 1 week or longer ago, perform a sensitive pregnancy test, and if it is negative she can receive an injection that day. If she has had unprotected sex after the 14 weeks and within the last 120 hours consider emergency contraception. She should be advised to use a backup method for 7 days. Asking her to return in 1 month if she has no menses is not necessary, as she may very likely not have periods (Hatcher et al., pp. 169, 172).

98. **(b)** The rolled rim of the condom should be on the outside. The condom should not be unrolled before it is placed on the penis. The penis should be removed from the vagina while it is still erect, and when completely away from her genitals, the condom should be removed. Condoms that are stored in a cool and dry place out of direct sunlight can be used up to 5 years past the manufacture date. (Hatcher et al., pp. 309–311).

99. **(a)** A contraceptive method such as the diaphragm requires that the user follow instructions correctly each time she has sexual intercourse. This is the reason that the typical failure rate (16%) for the diaphragm is significantly different than the perfect user failure (6%) rate. Intrauterine contraception (IUC), etonogestrel implant (Implanon), and tubal sterilization's effectiveness do not depend on having to follow instructions correctly with each intercourse. Typical and perfect use failure rates are the same or less than 1% different with these three methods (Hatcher et al., p. 24).

100. **(d)** Oral contraceptive use has been shown to decrease the risk for both ovarian and endometrial cancer (Hatcher et al., pp. 204–205).

101. **(c)** Normal semen analysis characteristics include a total sperm concentration > 20 million/mL, motility of > 50% with forward progression, and morphology > 30% normal (Gibbs et al., p. 707).

102. **(b)** This procedure, in addition to being used for evaluation of tubal patency, is in some cases also therapeutic. Postprocedure pregnancy rates are highest when an oil-based medium is used. HSG is performed ideally in the early to midfollicular phase. This timing reduces the risk of irradiating an existing pregnancy. In the procedure, radiopaque dye is injected via a cannula through the cervix. Two radiographic views are usually taken, to evaluate the uterus and fallopian tubes. (Gibbs et al., p. 708; Schuiling & Likis, p. 391).

103. **(a)** A varicocele is a dilatation of the internal spermatic vein. It is believed to cause infertility by raising the testicular temperature, which causes decreased sperm production (Schuiling & Likis, p. 386).

104. **(a)** Cervical mucus becomes clear, watery, and stretchy, resembling raw egg whites, under the influence of estrogen just prior to ovulation. When allowed to dry, it produces a fern pattern (Schuiling & Likis, p. 99).

105. **(d)** Studies have failed to confirm that moderate caffeine consumption (250 mg/day) by men or women has any negative impact on fertility. There is some evidence that higher levels of caffeine intake by women may delay conception or increase the risk of pregnancy loss. Cocaine use can impair spermatogenesis. Marijuana use can inhibit the secretion of GnRH and may suppress reproductive function in both women and men. Heavy alcohol use by both men and women may have a negative impact on fertility (Speroff & Fritz, p. 1023).

106. **(b)** Clomiphene citrate has both estrogen antagonist and agonist properties. However, it works primarily as an antagonist blocking estrogen receptors so that the normal ovarian-hypothalamic-estrogen feedback loop is altered. There is then an increase in GnRH release resulting in an increase in gonadotropin secretion (Speroff & Fritz, pp. 1177–1178).

107. **(c)** Pregnancy rates following a vasectomy reversal range from 38 to 89%. Success depends on the skill of the surgeon, the length of time since the vasectomy was performed, the presence of antisperm antibodies, the age of the female, and the location and length of the vas segment removed. There is no known increased risk of birth defects related to vasectomy reversal. Studies have indicated that until age 64 a man's age does not affect sperm or the ability to fertilize eggs (Hatcher et al., p. 391).

108. **(c)** Hot flashes occur in about 10% of women during use of clomiphene citrate. Mood swings are also common (Speroff & Fritz, p. 1181).

109. **(a)** Chlamydia, gonorrhea, trichomoniasis, and herpes cervicitis may all present with vaginal discharge, dysuria, postcoital bleeding, and cervical friability. The wet mount will demonstrate many WBCs. While she could have more than one infection, the differentiating piece of information is that gonorrhea is the only one of these infections caused by gram negative diplococcus (CDC, p. 35).

110. **(a)** The CDC recommended treatment regimen for uncomplicated gonorrhea in a nonpregnant female is ceftriaxone 125 mg IM in a single dose plus treatment for chlamydia if infection is not ruled out (CDC, p. 45).

111. **(d)** *Molluscum contagiosum* is caused by a virus. Lesions are typically dome shaped, waxy papules with central umbilications. They are usually 1 to 5 mm in size, flesh to white colored, and occur most commonly on the

trunk and anogenital region. They are not painful or pruritic. The lesions of acne vulgaris include open and closed comedones, inflammatory papules and pustules. Erythema nodosum presents as very tender lesions that are pink or red and are 1 to 10 cm in diameter. Folliculitis is an inflammatory reaction in a hair follicle characterized by a pustular lesion with central hair (Hatcher et al., p. 548).

112. **(a)** *Molluscum contagiosum* is a self-limiting infection often resolving spontaneously within a few months. If the infection is bothersome, cryotherapy with liquid nitrogen, trichloroacetic acid application, or curettage may be used for destruction of lesions (Hatcher et al., p. 548).

113. **(b)** Systemic symptoms such as malaise and low-grade fever may occur with a primary or initial herpes episode. Such symptoms are less likely with recurrent episodes. The risk of herpes transmission exists both during asymptomatic periods and when there are prodromal symptoms. Topical therapy with acyclovir is less effective than oral therapy. Pregnant women without signs or symptoms of genital herpes or its prodrome at the onset of labor may deliver vaginally. (CDC, pp. 17–20; Hatcher et al., pp. 538–540).

114. **(d)** Imiquimod 5% cream is a patient applied treatment for external genital warts. It is applied once daily at bedtime, three times a week for up to 16 weeks. The area should be washed with soap and water 6 to 10 hours after medication application. The safety of imiquimod use during pregnancy has not been established. No data support the use of more than one type of treatment at a time to improve efficacy of treatment (CDC, pp. 64–65).

115. **(d)** The Jarisch-Herxheimer reaction is an acute febrile reaction with headache and myalgia that may occur within 24 hours after any therapy for syphilis. It occurs most commonly in individuals with early syphilis. Antipyretics may be recommended for symptomatic relief. It is not an allergic reaction to medication. There is no proven method to prevent this adverse reaction (CDC, pp. 23–24).

116. **(c)** The RPR (and VDRL) are nontreponemal tests. It is expected that these tests will eventually become nonreactive after treatment. The FTA-ABS and MHA-TP are both treponemal tests. Most individuals who have had syphilis will have a positive treponemal test for the remainder of their lives. There are exceptions for both of the above but they are just that— exceptions rather than the normal expected findings (CDC, p. 23).

117. **(d)** According to the CDC, empiric treatment of PID should be initiated in sexually active young women and others at risk for STDs if they have pelvic or lower abdominal pain, no other cause for the illness can be identified, and one or more of the following is present on pelvic examination: uterine tenderness, adnexal tenderness, or cervical motion tenderness (CDC, p. 57).

118. **(b)** A positive Darkfield examination of lesion exudate is diagnostic of primary syphilis. The CDC recommended treatment for primary syphilis is benzathine penicillin G 2.4 million units IM in a single dose (CDC, pp. 22–24).

119. **(a)** Vaginal candidiasis presents with vaginal itching and discharge, dyspareunia, vulvar dysuria, and vaginal burning, irritation, and soreness. Diagnostic findings include a normal pH of less than 4.5, negative amine,

and a wet mount showing no clue cells, few WBCs, and the presence of hyphae, pseudohyphae, buds, or filaments. Treatment will be with an antifungal agent such as terconazole. In bacterial vaginosis, the pH is greater than 4.5, amine is positive, and a wet mount will demonstrate clue cells and decreased lactobacilli. Trichomoniasis will demonstrate a pH of greater than 4.5, amine may be positive, and a wet mount will demonstrate many WBCs and motile trichomonads (Katz, et al., p. 589).

120. **(c)** The currently available treatments for genital warts do not eradicate the virus. The CDC currently recommends that treatment of partners is not necessary for the management of genital warts. An increase in the frequency of Pap tests is not recommended. If genital warts are located on the cervix, a Pap test should be done to assess for high grade squamous intraepithelial lesions prior to treatment (CDC, pp. 62–66).

121. **(a)** *Haemophilus ducreyi* is the causative organism in chancroid. The appearance of a painful genital ulcer and tender inguinal lymphadenopathy suggests a diagnosis of chancroid. When the above findings are accompanied by a suppurative inguinal adenopathy (bubo) the diagnosis of chancroid is almost certain (CDC, p. 15).

122. **(d)** Trichomoniasis usually presents with a foul smelling vaginal discharge and itching. Dysuria and dyspareunia may also be present. Examination findings include presence of a frothy, yellow-green vaginal discharge and vulvovaginal erythema. Petechial lesions may also be seen on the cervix and are sometimes called strawberry marks. Male partners are usually asymptomatic, but may have

symptoms of urethritis or prostatitis (CDC, p. 52; Hatcher et al., p. 552).

■ REFERENCES

American College of Obstetricians and Gynecologists (ACOG). (2009). Cervical cytology screening. *Practice Bulletin No. 109.* Washington, DC: Author.

American College of Obstetricians and Gynecologists (ACOG). (2008). Management of abnormal cervical cytology and histology. *Practice Bulletin No. 99.* Washington, DC: Author.

Buttaro, T., Trybulski, J., Bailey, P., & Sandberg-Cook, J. (2008). *Primary care: A collaborative practice* (3rd ed.). St. Louis, MO: Mosby, Inc.

Centers for Disease Control and Prevention (CDC). (2006). Sexually transmitted diseases treatment guidelines. *Morbidity and Mortality Weekly Report, 55*(RR-11).

Gibbs, R., Karlan, B., Haney, A., & Nygaard, I. (2008). *Danforth's obstetrics and gynecology* (10th ed.). Philadelphia, PA: Lippincott, Williams, & Wilkins.

Hatcher, R., Trussell, J., Nelson, A. et al. (2007). *Contraceptive technology* (19th ed.). New York, NY: Ardent Media.

Katz, V., Lentz, G., Lobo, R., & Gershenson, D. (2007). *Comprehensive gynecology* (5th ed.). Philadelphia, PA: Mosby Elsevier.

Lowdermilk, D., & Perry, S. (2007). *Maternity and women's health care* (9th ed.). St. Louis, MO: Mosby, Inc.

National Osteoporosis Foundation (NOF). (2008). *Clinician's guide to prevention and treatment of osteoporosis.* Washington, DC: Author.

North American Menopause Society (NAMS). (2007). *Menopause practice: A clinician's guide* (3rd ed.). Cleveland, OH: Author.

Schuiling, K., & Likis, F. (2006). *Women's gynecologic health.* Sudbury, MA: Jones and Bartlett.

Seidel, H., Ball, J., Dains, J., & Benedict, G. (2006). *Mosby's guide to physical examination* (6th ed.). St. Louis, MO: Mosby, Inc.

Smith, R., Cokkinides, V., & Brawley, O. (2008). Cancer screening in the United States: A review of current American Cancer Society guidelines and cancer screening issues. *CA Cancer Journal for Clinicians, 58*, 161–179.

Speroff, L., & Fritz, M. (2005). *Clinical gynecologic endocrinology and infertility* (7th ed). Philadelphia, PA: Lippincott, Williams, & Wilkins.

US Department of Justice Office on Violence Against Women. (2004). *A national protocol for sexual assault medical forensic examinations: Adults and adolescents.* Washington, DC: Author.

Wynne, A., Woo, T., & Olyaei, A. (2007). *Pharmacotherapuetics for nurse practitioner subscribers* (2nd ed.). Philadelphia, PA: F. A. Davis Company.

3

Obstetrics

Beth M. Kelsey

Anne Salomone

Select one best answer to the following questions.

1. A common discomfort in pregnancy that may occur as a result of increased progesterone levels is:

   a. Constipation
   b. Gum bleeding
   c. Low back pain
   d. Nasal stuffiness

2. A pregnant woman is 5'6" in height and has a prepregnancy weight of 130 lbs. Which of the following would represent the most appropriate weight for her by the end of her pregnancy?

   a. 145 lbs
   b. 150 lbs
   c. 165 lbs
   d. 170 lbs

3. A client presents for her first prenatal visit. She had discontinued DMPA about 8 months ago and has not had a period for about a year. She denies feeling any fetal movement. Fundal height is half way between the symphysis and umbilicus. Your initial as-

sessment of her gestation given this information is that she is:

   a. 12 weeks pregnant
   b. 16 weeks pregnant
   c. 20 weeks pregnant
   d. 24 weeks pregnant

4. Relief from heartburn during pregnancy may be obtained by:

   a. Drinking a large glass of water with meals
   b. Eating 5 or 6 small meals each day
   c. Lying down for 30 minutes after meals
   d. Taking an antacid with her iron supplement

5. A woman presents with the complaints of no menses for 3 months, nausea, breast tenderness, and urinary frequency. She believes she is pregnant. These symptoms are classified as:

   a. Presumptive indicators of pregnancy
   b. Probable indicators of pregnancy
   c. Positive indicators of pregnancy
   d. Objective indicators of pregnancy

6. Upon auscultating the heart of a pregnant woman who is at 16 weeks' gestation, you notice that she has a split S_1. Appropriate management would include:

   a. Advising her to limit her physical activity
   b. Reevaluating her heart in the third trimester
   c. Recognizing that this is a normal finding
   d. Scheduling an echocardiogram

7. A woman is currently pregnant and has had three full term deliveries. One of these babies died at 4 months from SIDS. She has also had one stillbirth at 34 weeks and one spontaneous abortion. Using the terminology of gravida (G), term (T), preterm (P), abortion (A), living (L), which of the following correctly represents her pregnancy history?

   a. G5 T4 P0 A1 L3
   b. G5 T3 P1 A1 L2
   c. G6 T3 P0 A2 L3
   d. G6 T3 P1 A1 L2

8. Human chorionic gonadotropin (hCG) is produced by the:

   a. Corpus luteum
   b. Fetus
   c. Pituitary gland
   d. Trophoblast

9. Which thyroid hormone remains within nonpregnant normal limits during pregnancy?

   a. TSH
   b. Total T_4
   c. TBG
   d. Total T_3

10. Using Naegele's rule, the estimated date of delivery (EDD) for a pregnant woman with an LMP of November 20 would be:

    a. August 6
    b. August 13
    c. August 20
    d. August 27

11. A PPD test is done as part of routine screening for a 14-weeks-pregnant client who has no risk factors for tuberculosis. The test is positive with an induration of 15 mm. Management for this client should include:

    a. Obtaining a chest radiograph after delivery
    b. Obtaining a chest radiograph now
    c. Immediate initiation of isoniazid
    d. Initiation of isoniazid after delivery

12. CDC guidelines for HIV screening of pregnant women include:

    a. Counseling all pregnant women that it is important to have HIV screen in early third trimester
    b. Performing risk factor assessment and screening women based on risks for HIV infection
    c. Screening all pregnant women for HIV in the first and third trimesters
    d. Screening all pregnant women for HIV as early in pregnancy as possible unless they decline testing

13. A client presents for a routine visit at 24 weeks' gestation. She relates that she has discontinued taking her prenatal vitamins as she believes they are making the skin around her eyes and face darken. You advise her that:

    a. She should change to a supplement that does not contain iron
    b. This may be due to a hereditary type of anemia
    c. Getting some sun exposure will help to even out the color
    d. The darker pigmentation usually fades after the baby is born

14. The hormone human placental lactogen (hPL):

    a. Stimulates the growth of the breasts and has lactogenic properties

b. Causes a relaxation of the joints resulting in the "waddle" of pregnancy

c. Promotes the development of oxytocin receptors in the cervix

d. Causes vasodilation and the drop in blood pressure seen in the second trimester

15. Expected pelvic examination findings at 8 weeks' gestation include:

a. Braxton Hicks contractions
b. Dextrorotation of the uterus
c. Softening of the uterine isthmus
d. Uterus palpable at the symphysis pubis

16. Which of the following may occur as a result of normal changes in the renal system during pregnancy?

a. Decrease in glomerular filtration rate
b. Decrease in sodium excretion
c. Increase in creatinine levels
d. Increase in urine glucose

17. Hemodynamic changes that occur during pregnancy include:

a. Decrease in heart rate and red blood cell mass
b. Increase in cardiac output and blood volume
c. Slight increase in systolic blood pressure in second trimester
d. Slight decrease in white blood cell count in third trimester

18. Results of a urine culture from a clean catch urine specimen obtained at an initial prenatal visit indicate the presence of 50,000 *E. coli* per mL of urine. The client currently has no urinary complaints. Appropriate management would include:

a. Instructing the client that no treatment is needed at this time but to report any urinary tract infection symptoms
b. Repeating the urine culture to assure that the results were not due to contamination

c. Initiating antibiotic therapy and repeating the urine culture 2 weeks after treatment is completed
d. Initiating suppressive therapy and checking urine at each visit for nitrites or leukocyte esterase

19. A 32-weeks-pregnant client complains of frequent leg cramps. She currently walks 30 minutes each day for exercise. Interventions to decrease this client's leg cramps would include:

a. Alternately flexing and extending the feet
b. Decreasing the amount of daily walking
c. Increasing the amount of magnesium in her diet
d. Taking a daily phosphorus supplement

20. Folic acid supplementation prior to conception has been shown to decrease the incidence of:

a. Cardiac anomalies
b. Down syndrome
c. Neural tube defects
d. Spontaneous abortion

21. In the preembryonic stage, the inner cell mass called the blastocyst will eventually become the:

a. Yolk sac, amnion, and placenta
b. Second polar body
c. Embryo, amnion, and yolk sac membrane
d. Maternal side of the chorion and placenta

22. The gestational age at greatest risk for taking a drug that can cause cardiac anomalies is:

a. 1 to 3 weeks
b. 3 to 8 weeks
c. 8 to 11 weeks
d. 11 to 14 weeks

23. The corpus luteum is responsible for secreting:

    a. hCG to maintain the pregnancy during the first trimester
    b. Progesterone to maintain the uterine lining for implantation
    c. Human placental lactogen to promote placental formation
    d. Prolactin to promote growth of the ductal system of the breasts

24. A woman who is currently pregnant and has had two miscarriages would be considered a:

    a. Multipara
    b. Nulligravida
    c. Nullipara
    d. Primigravida

25. A 10-weeks-pregnant woman has stepped on a rusty piece of metal requiring several stitches to close the laceration. Her last tetanus injection was 10 years ago. Appropriate advice would include telling her that:

    a. She should not receive the tetanus booster while she is in her first trimester.
    b. If she received a complete primary series of three injections a booster is not needed.
    c. The tetanus vaccine is a toxoid and is considered safe to give during pregnancy.
    d. Tetanus immune globulin should be given rather than a booster vaccination.

26. A frantic client calls your office today. She is at 28 weeks' gestation and her husband has just been diagnosed with varicella zoster (VZV). She thinks she had chicken pox when she was a child. You advise her that she should:

    a. Receive (varicella zoster immunoglobulin) VZIG
    b. Start oral acyclovir now
    c. Have a VZV immunoglobulin G (IgG) level checked as soon as possible
    d. Have a targeted ultrasound to check the fetus for signs of infection

27. Amniocentesis may be used in the assessment of:

    a. Amniotic embolism
    b. Amniotic fluid volume
    c. Fetal lung maturity
    d. Placental blood flow

28. By definition, a reactive NST demonstrates:

    a. A minimum of 2 or more accelerations in the fetal heart rate of 10 beats or more, for 10 or more seconds, in a 10-minute period
    b. Two or more decelerations in the fetal heart rate of 10 or more beats, for 10 or more seconds, in a 10-minute period
    c. A minimum of 2 or more accelerations in the fetal heart rate of 15 or more beats, for 15 or more seconds, in a 20-minute period
    d. A minimum of 4 or more accelerations in the fetal heart rate of 15 or more beats, for 15 or more seconds, in a 15-minute period

29. During an ultrasound examination, a 32-week-pregnant woman states that she is feeling dizzy and lightheaded. She is diaphoretic and pale. This woman is most likely experiencing:

    a. An anxiety attack
    b. Hypoglycemia
    c. Orthostatic hypotension
    d. Vena cava syndrome

30. The result of a biophysical profile (BPP) performed at 36 weeks' gestation reveals a score of 6 including a normal amniotic fluid volume. Counseling for this client should include that:

    a. The biophysical profile will need to be repeated in one week.
    b. She will probably have a contraction stress test scheduled.
    c. Nonstress tests will be scheduled twice weekly until delivery.
    d. Delivery may be considered at this time if the fetus is mature.

31. Instructions on monitoring fetal activity for a pregnant woman who is at 32 weeks' gestation should include which of the following?

    a. Expect a noticeable decrease in movement as the pregnancy nears term.
    b. There should be at least 10 movements identified in a 12-hour period.
    c. Plan to monitor fetal movement daily after a meal when the fetus will be most active.
    d. Vary the time of day for counting to ensure an adequate assessment.

32. A 38-weeks-pregnant diabetic client is being evaluated for possible induction of labor because of concerns about macrosomia. In determining the chances for a successful induction, Bishop's scoring is done. The components of this scoring include evaluation for:

    a. Cervical consistency
    b. Loss of the mucus plug
    c. Position of the fetus
    d. Rupture of membranes

Questions 33 and 34 refer to the following monitor strip:

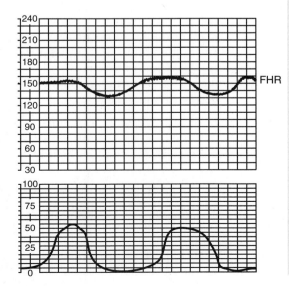

33. The most likely cause of the type of the decelerations seen on the above monitor strip is:

    a. Fetal sleep cycling
    b. Head compression
    c. Umbilical cord compression
    d. Uteroplacental insufficiency

34. A laboring woman, whose only medication has been meperidine hydrochloride 50 mg IM, has the above monitor strip reading. Management for this woman would include:

    a. Administering an opiate antagonist such as naloxone
    b. Continuing routine care and fetal heart rate monitoring
    c. Performing a vaginal examination to assess for a prolapsed cord
    d. Turning her on her left side and administering oxygen

35. A 36-weeks-pregnant client with possible intrauterine growth retardation (IUGR) has a negative contraction stress test. The most likely intervention will be:

    a. Follow-up with a biophysical profile
    b. Immediate delivery by C-section
    c. Repeating the test in 24 to 48 hours
    d. Repeating the test in 1 week

36. The following is recorded as findings from a vaginal examination of a laboring woman with a fetus in vertex position: 50%, 3 cm, −1. Which of the following would be a correct interpretation of this data?

    a. Dilatation of the cervix is 50% complete
    b. The cervix length is 3 centimeters
    c. The fetal head is above the ischial spines
    d. The fetal presenting part is floating

37. A client presents with a positive urine hCG and last normal menstrual period (LNMP) 6 weeks ago. She states she has had a small amount of

bright red vaginal bleeding for the past 12 hours. She is also having mild abdominal cramping pain. A pelvic examination reveals a closed cervix, small amount of bright red blood at the cervical os and a slightly enlarged uterus. The differential diagnosis for this woman includes:

a. Ectopic pregnancy and inevitable abortion
b. Ectopic pregnancy and threatened abortion
c. Implantation bleeding and threatened abortion
d. Inevitable abortion and incomplete abortion

38. Suggested high iron foods for the vegetarian pregnant woman who does consume dairy products include:

a. Beans and lentils
b. Canola oil
c. Cheese and yogurt
d. Peanut butter

39. The CDC's recommended management of condyloma acuminata during pregnancy is:

a. Application of podophyllin to external condyloma only
b. Application of trichloroacetic acid to condyloma
c. Application of imiquimod 5% cream to condyloma
d. Delay of any treatment until after delivery

40. A pregnant woman who is at 36 weeks' gestation presents with complaint of an occasional trickle of fluid from her vagina for the past 6 hours. She is not having any contractions. When testing the pH of the fluid to assess for premature rupture of membranes you will want to remember that:

a. A swab should be used to obtain the specimen because speculum exam is contraindicated.
b. Amniotic fluid should have a pH of 6.0 or less.

c. Vaginal infection should not interfere with interpreting the pH.
d. You should ask her if she has had sexual intercourse in the past several hours.

41. A couple presents for genetic counseling. They are both autosomal recessive for sickle cell anemia. You can tell them that their risk for having an infant born with sickle cell disease is:

a. 1 in 4 chance (25%)
b. 2 in 4 chance (50%)
c. 4 in 4 chance (100%)
d. No chance (0%)

42. Which of the following is correct concerning screening pregnant women for Group B strepococcus?

a. All pregnant women should be screened between 35 and 37 weeks' gestation.
b. Cultures should be obtained from both the cervix and rectum.
c. Treatment with antibiotics should be initiated immediately if culture is positive.
d. Women with risk factors should be screened each trimester.

43. Which of the following statements concerning chorionic villi sampling is true?

a. Both chromosomal and DNA information can be obtained.
b. The test is useful in the early diagnosis of neural tube defects.
c. The test is ideally performed prior to 10 weeks' gestation.
d. Pregnancy loss rates are higher than with amniocentesis.

44. Which of the following pregnant clients would be most at risk for intrauterine growth retardation (IUGR)?

a. 17 year old, G1 P0 with a Hgb of 11.8 at 30 weeks
b. 24 year old, G2 P1 with a previous preterm birth
c. 28 year old, G1 P0 with chronic hypertension
d. 32 year old, G2 P1 with BMI of 30

45. A 26-weeks-pregnant Rh negative client is in an automobile accident and fetomaternal hemorrhage is suspected. Which of the following tests would be used to determine the dose of Rh-immune globulin to be given to this client?

    a. Direct Coombs
    b. Indirect Coombs
    c. Kliehauer-Betke
    d. Rh antibody titer

46. One treatment for ectopic pregnancy is the use of methotrexate. This drug works by:

    a. Stopping the growth of the corpus luteum
    b. Increasing the peristalsis of the fallopian tube
    c. Inhibiting DNA synthesis and cell multiplication
    d. Causing a disruption of the endometrium

47. Which of the following supplements should be avoided during treatment for ectopic pregnancy with methotrexate?

    a. Calcium
    b. Folic acid
    c. Iron
    d. Vitamin B$_{12}$

48. A 28-year-old client is being seen for her initial prenatal visit at 10 weeks' gestation. She states she is used to running a distance of 5 miles four to five times a week and wants to know if she can continue this exercise routine. The most appropriate response would be to tell this client that:

    a. She should enroll in an aerobics class as there is less risk of muscle injury.
    b. She should walk to decrease the risk for fetal hyperthermia.
    c. She can continue to run but should decrease the frequency to 2 to 3 times a week.
    d. She should monitor her weight gain to assure she is getting adequate calories.

Questions 49 and 50 refer to the following scenario.

A 40-year-old G1 P0 at 32 weeks' gestation presents with bright red vaginal bleeding for the past 6 hours, back pain, and irregular, abdominal cramping. Her pregnancy has been complicated by chronic hypertension. Examination reveals diffuse abdominal tenderness and increased uterine tone. Vital signs are unchanged from previous visits.

49. Given this information, you suspect:

    a. Marginal placenta previa
    b. Hemorrhagic cystitis
    c. HELLP syndrome
    d. Placental abruption

50. The immediate plan of care for this client in addition to obtaining a CBC and blood type with crossmatch, should include:

    a. Continuous fetal monitoring, urinalysis, and CT scan of the pelvis
    b. Chemistry profile, 24-hour urine for protein and creatinine clearance, and intermittent fetal monitoring
    c. Ultrasound, intermittent fetal monitoring, and 24-hour urine for protein and creatinine clearance
    d. Ultrasound, continuous fetal monitoring, and coagulation studies

51. Increased risk for placental abruption has been associated with:

    a. Cocaine use
    b. Diabetes
    c. Obesity
    d. Pyelonephritis

52. HELLP syndrome stands for:

    a. Hypertension, elevated leukocytes, low platelets
    b. Hypertension, elevated liver enzymes, lethargy, proteinuria
    c. Hemolysis, elevated liver enzymes, low platelets
    d. Hemolysis, elevated leukocytes, lethargy, proteinuria

53. At 16 weeks' gestation a woman has a BP of 142/92 with the same reading when repeated 6 hours later. At 28 weeks she has a BP of 148/98 and 2+ proteinuria. At this time her diagnosis would be:

    a. Chronic hypertension
    b. Idiopathic hypertension
    c. Mild preeclampsia superimposed on chronic hypertension
    d. Severe preeclampsia

54. Risk factors for asymptomatic bacteriuria in pregnancy include:

    a. Multiple pregnancies
    b. Premature labor
    c. Hypertension
    d. Sickle cell disease

55. Which of the following is not a normal change in glucose metabolism during pregnancy?

    a. Decrease in insulin production related to insulin-antagonist effects of placental hormones
    b. Increase in fetal nutrient needs and glucose use in late pregnancy
    c. Increase in maternal insulin resistance because of insulin-antagonistic effects of placental hormones
    d. Increase in insulin production to compensate for insulin resistance

56. The recommended time schedule for routine gestational diabetes screening is:

    a. Whenever the initial prenatal laboratory tests are performed
    b. With initial prenatal laboratory tests and at 28 weeks
    c. Between 24 and 28 weeks of gestation
    d. Each trimester if the woman has diabetes risk factors

57. A diagnosis of gestational diabetes is made when:

    a. The 1-hour plasma value is 150 mg
    b. One or more values on plasma samples are exceeded: Fasting—105 mg, 1 hour—190 mg, 2 hour—165 mg, 3 hour—145 mg
    c. Two or more values on plasma samples are exceeded: Fasting—105 mg, 1 hour—190 mg, 2 hour—165 mg, 3 hour—145 mg
    d. Three or more values on plasma samples are exceeded: Fasting—120 mg, 1 hour—145 mg, 2 hour—130 mg, 3 hour—110 mg

58. A woman with diabetes who would like to become pregnant has come to the office for preconception counseling. She currently takes regular and NPH insulin twice a day. Counseling for this client should include the following information:

    a. A glycosylated hemoglobin level should be obtained prior to conception.
    b. She will need to change to an oral hypoglycemic prior to conception.
    c. She will probably need to increase her insulin dosage in the first trimester.
    d. Strict glucose control prior to conception will prevent fetal macrosomia.

59. A 28-year-old pregnant woman presents for her initial prenatal visit. She is healthy except for mild persistent asthma. She currently uses the low-dose inhaled corticosteroid, budesonide, on a daily basis and the short-acting inhaled beta-2 agonist, albuterol, as needed. Education concerning management of her asthma during pregnancy should include:

    a. Exacerbations are common during labor and delivery.
    b. She may continue her current medications and monitor for any needed changes.

c. She will need to switch to theo-phylline as the inhaled cortico-steroids are contraindicated during pregnancy.
d. She will not be able to use her beta-2 agonist when breastfeeding.

60. A 39-weeks-pregnant client presents with a mild sore throat and nasal congestion. Her temperature is 99.8°F. Appropriate relief measures would include:

a. Aspirin and increase fluid intake
b. Acetaminophen and a nasal de-congestant spray
c. Ibuprofen and salt water gargles
d. Naproxen and pseudoephedrine

61. An Rh negative pregnant woman should be given Rho (D) immune globulin (RhoGAM) after delivery if she has a:

a. Negative indirect Coombs test and the baby is Rh negative
b. Positive indirect Coombs test and the baby is Rh negative
c. Negative indirect Coombs test and the baby is Rh positive
d. Positive indirect Coombs test and the baby is Rh positive

62. A blood antibody screen demonstrates a Kell antibody. You know that Kell:

a. Isoimmunization can occur and can produce erythroblastosis fetalis
b. Antibodies are associated with a recent viral illness and are insignificant
c. Is from a prior transfusion and is not significant to the fetus but will make it more difficult to find a crossmatch for the mother
d. Antibody formation can be prevented by administering RhoGAM

63. There would be a risk for fetal ABO hemolytic disease if a mother who was:

a. Type A, delivered an infant who was type O
b. Type B, delivered an infant who was type O
c. Type O, delivered an infant who was type A
d. Type AB, delivered an infant who was type O

64. A Liley graph (optical density graph) is used in Rh-sensitized pregnancies to assess the risk to the fetus of an adverse outcome by plotting:

a. The mother's antibody titers
b. Amniotic fluid bilirubin levels
c. Fetal hemoglobin levels
d. Predictive ultrasound parameters

65. A 25-year-old primiparous woman who is at 17 weeks' gestation is being seen today for a routine antepartum visit. She is scheduled to have a maternal serum alpha-fetoprotein (MSAFP) drawn at this visit. She now states that she is not sure that she wants this test done because several of her friends had the test come back "abnormal." They worried the whole pregnancy that something was wrong with their babies, but all were born normal. In counseling her, you:

a. Acknowledge her fear, and explain that false positives only occur if gestational dates are inaccurate
b. Explain that the MSAFP test is a screening test and only indicates individuals who may warrant further testing
c. Explain that the test is usually repeated in 4 to 8 weeks if the initial results are abnormal
d. Advise her that she can cancel the test today and reschedule it any-time if she decides that she does want it

66. The most common preventable type of birth defect in the United States is:

a. Neural tube defect
b. Fetal alcohol syndrome

c. Intrauterine growth retardation
d. Down syndrome

67. A 28-year-old G1 P0 client presents for her first prenatal visit. You find that she has a history of genital herpes and a lesion on her labia minora. She relates she has one to two outbreaks a year. You counsel her that:

a. Prophylactic therapy with acyclovir is recommended after the first trimester to prevent perinatal transmission.
b. She will need Cesarean delivery to prevent perinatal transmission.
c. She will need to have a careful perineal examination when she presents for delivery and if no lesions are present she can have a vaginal delivery.
d. She will need serial cervical cultures for HSV starting at 32 weeks. If any are positive she will need a Cesarean delivery.

68. Asymmetric intrauterine growth restriction (IUGR) would be most likely to occur when:

a. The mother smokes cigarettes
b. The mother has severe preeclampsia
c. The fetus has cardiovascular anomalies
d. There is more than one fetus

69. TORCH titer stands for:

a. Toxoplasmosis; Oral herpes; Rubella; Chlamydia; Herpes simplex
b. Toxoplasmosis; Oral herpes; Rubella; Chlamydia; Hepatitis
c. Toxoplasmosis; Other infections; Rubella; Cytomegalovirus; Herpes simplex
d. Toxoplasmosis; Other infections; Rubella; Cytomegalovirus; Hepatitis

70. A woman is exposed to human parvovirus (fifth disease) during the 24th week of gestation. You know that:

a. Fetal infection is likely and there is a high chance of preterm labor or stillbirth.
b. Less than 50% of pregnant women are immune to this infection.
c. The risk of infection after exposure in susceptible women is about 50%.
d. The viral load will determine if there is concern over a problem for the fetus.

71. Polyhydramnios is associated with:

a. Maternal hypertension
b. Neural tube defects
c. Postterm pregnancy
d. Pulmonary hypoplasia

72. A fetal anomaly that would increase the likelihood of oligohydramnios is:

a. Esophageal atresia
b. Hydrocephalus
c. Renal agenesis
d. Meningomyelocele

73. A woman with current deep vein thrombosis confirmed by Doppler studies would meet the criteria for a diagnosis of antiphospholipid syndrome (APS) if she also had:

a. At least one other thrombotic event not related to injury
b. Presence of lupus anticoagulant on two or more occasions at least 6 weeks apart
c. Three or more unexplained consecutive spontaneous abortions before the 10th week of gestation
d. An unexplained death of a normal fetus at or beyond the 10th week of gestation

74. You are giving your near-term patient instructions on when to go to the hospital. You tell her that true labor contractions should be regular and should be timed from the:

a. Beginning of one contraction to the beginning of the next contraction

b. End of one contraction to the beginning of the next contraction

c. End of one contraction to the end of the next contraction

d. Peak of one contraction to the peak of the next contraction

75. A second degree laceration involves the vaginal mucosa:

a. Posterior fourchette, and perineal skin

b. Posterior fourchette, periurethral area, and perineal skin

c. Posterior fourchette, perineal skin, and perineal muscles

d. Periurethral area, perineal skin, and external anal sphincter

76. First stage of labor is defined as lasting from the onset of:

a. Contractions until active cervical dilatation occurs

b. Regular contractions with cervical change until transition

c. Regular contractions with cervical change until complete dilatation

d. Cervical change until the delivery of the infant

77. During a routine antepartum visit your patient asks what the usual monitoring procedure is for the baby during labor. Since she has no identified risks you advise her that the usual guidelines for monitoring fetal heart rate in labor are:

a. To check the FHR at least every 30 minutes during the first stage of active labor and every 15 minutes during the second stage of labor

b. Continuous fetal monitoring after the cervix has dilated to 8 cm or membranes have ruptured

c. To check the FHR every hour during the first stage of active labor, every 30 minutes during transition, and every 15 minutes during the second stage of labor

d. Continuous fetal monitoring whenever the patient is in bed but can be discontinued whenever she wants to get up to walk

78. What is the normal mechanism for labor in a vertex presentation?

a. Descent, engagement, internal rotation, flexion, external rotation, extension

b. Engagement, descent, internal rotation, flexion, extension, external rotation

c. Internal rotation, engagement, descent, extension, flexion, external rotation

d. Engagement, descent, flexion, internal rotation, extension, external rotation

79. A 27-year-old G2 P1 had a C-section with her last delivery because of a transverse lie. She relates that they told her that the baby was "stuck" in the top of her uterus and they had to "do an extra little cut up there" to get him out. She is interested in having a vaginal birth after Cesarean section (VBAC) with this pregnancy. You tell her that:

a. She is probably a candidate for a VBAC if the baby is less than 4000 g.

b. She may not be a candidate for a VBAC assuming the medical records confirm her story.

c. As long as she does not require pitocin, she should be able to have a VBAC.

d. As long as the fetus is not in a transverse lie, she should be able to have a VBAC.

80. A 25-year-old G1 P0 at 38 weeks' gestation has had an uncomplicated pregnancy. She presents today for a routine visit. She relates that the baby was extremely active yesterday but has not moved today. She states she is having a few contractions and lost her mucus plug 4 days ago. Given this information you:

a. Recognize that it is common to have the baby stop moving shortly before labor

b. Are concerned that there is a problem because of the lack of fetal movement
c. Recognize that labor is imminent as she has lost her mucus plug
d. Do a sterile speculum examination to check for ruptured membranes

81. In a woman who has been diagnosed with an intrauterine fetal demise (IUFD):

a. Delivery should be induced as soon as possible to reduce the risk for intrauterine infection.
b. Parents should be offered the option of labor induction or waiting for spontaneous labor.
c. Waiting for spontaneous labor allows the parents to have a more healthy grieving process.
d. There is a high risk for maternal coagulopathy within the first week after fetal demise.

82. Complications associated with post-term pregnancy include:

a. Macrosomia, meconium aspiration, polyhydramnios
b. Growth retardation, preeclampsia, oligohydramnios
c. Macrosomia, increased risk for C-section delivery, placental insufficiency
d. Preeclampsia, meconium aspiration, oligohydramnios

83. A 16-year-old client who is at 37 weeks' gestation is admitted to the hospital with severe preeclampsia. Magnesium sulfate ($MgSO_4$) is ordered. The primary reason for administering $MgSO_4$ to this client is to:

a. Increase urinary output
b. Lower blood pressure
c. Prevent seizure activity
d. Promote uterine relaxation

84. During assessment of the client on $MgSO_4$, a sign of developing toxicity would be:

a. Headache with blurred vision
b. Increased deep tendon reflexes
c. Severe right upper quadrant pain
d. Urinary output less than 30 mL/hr

85. The antidote for $MgSO_4$ toxicity is:

a. Betamethasone
b. Calcium gluconate
c. Nifedipine
d. Propranolol

86. A 40-year-old woman presents for her initial prenatal visit 14 weeks from her LNMP. She is complaining of severe nausea with vomiting and some vaginal spotting. On examination her fundus is at the umbilicus and there are no fetal heart tones. The most likely diagnosis for this woman is:

a. Hydatidiform mole
b. Missed abortion
c. Multiple gestation
d. Polyhydramnios

87. The hormone responsible for the letdown reflex during lactation is:

a. Estrogen
b. Progesterone
c. Prolactin
d. Oxytocin

88. A 36-year-old primipara presents with her LNMP at 14 weeks ago. She complains of fatigue, backache, and nausea and vomiting all day. Her vital signs and physical examination are within normal limits. Fundal height is two fingerbreadths below the umbilicus. Fetal heart tones are present. Routine prenatal laboratory tests are ordered. Other prenatal care for this client should include:

a. Scheduling her to return in 1 to 2 weeks for an MSAFP
b. Obtaining an MSAFP at this visit and having her return in 4 weeks
c. Scheduling an ultrasound and ordering a quantitative hCG
d. Scheduling her for an ultrasound as soon as possible

89. Potential complications for twin gestation include:

    a. Preterm labor, hyperemesis, and gestational diabetes
    b. Cord accidents, congenital anomalies, and thrombophlebitis
    c. Congenital anomalies, placental abruption, and postpartum hemorrhage
    d. Anemia, thrombophlebitis, cord accidents, and gallstones

90. Healthy twins, one girl and one boy, are delivered at 36 weeks' gestation. You send the placenta to pathology. What report would you expect to get back?

    a. Monochorionic-monoamniotic
    b. Monochorionic-diamniotic
    c. Dichorionic-diamniotic
    d. Dichorionic-monoamniotic

Questions 91, 92, and 93 refer to the following scenario.

An 18-year-old pregnant client who has received no prenatal care presents to the labor and delivery unit on August 6th contracting every 5 minutes for 50 seconds. The contractions are moderate to strong to palpation. She states that her last period was "for sure" on New Year's Day. Fundal height is 31 cm with the fetus in the vertex position. A nonstress test is reactive.

91. The next assessment that should be done is a:

    a. Biophysical profile
    b. Sterile digital examination
    c. Sterile speculum examination
    d. Transvaginal ultrasound

92. During assessment of this client several genital specimens were obtained. The test that requires a specimen from the posterior vaginal fornix or external cervical os is the:

    a. Fern pattern test
    b. Fibronectin assay
    c. Nitrazine pH test
    d. Group B streptococcus culture

93. A decision has been made to initiate tocolytic therapy. Betamethasone IM is also administered. This is done because administration of corticosteroids:

    a. Decreases possible respiratory side-effects of tocolytic drugs
    b. Decreases the incidence of premature rupture of membranes
    c. Enhances the ability of tocolytics to prolong pregnancy
    d. Reduces the incidence of newborn respiratory distress syndrome

94. The tocolytic agent terbutaline is administered to stop preterm labor. Maternal complications with this medication include:

    a. Pulmonary edema
    b. Hypertension
    c. Respiratory depression
    d. Severe bronchospasms

95. On examining a woman who had a normal spontaneous vaginal delivery 10 hours ago you would expect to find the fundus:

    a. At the umbilicus, the vagina gaping, and bright red bleeding on the perineal pad
    b. Three quarters of the way between the symphysis and umbilicus, the vagina edematous, and bright red bleeding on the perineal pad
    c. 1 to 2 fingerbreadths above the umbilicus, the vagina gaping, and serous vaginal bleeding on the pad
    d. 1 to 2 fingerbreadths below the umbilicus, the vagina edematous, and serous vaginal bleeding on the pad

96. 16 hours after a normal spontaneous vaginal delivery, a breastfeeding woman has a WBC count of 20,000 mm³. She also has a temperature of

100.2°F. Initial management would include:

a. Apply warm compresses to breasts
b. Encourage adequate fluids and rest
c. Order a transvaginal ultrasound
d. Order urinalysis and urine culture

97. For the woman who chooses not to breast feed, advice on enhancing suppression of lactation and decreasing discomfort would include:

a. Applying warm compresses to the breasts every 4 hours
b. Considering the use of prolactin inhibiting medication
c. Avoiding wearing a brassiere as this will stimulate the nipples
d. Avoiding letting shower water flow over the breasts

98. Which of the following contraceptive methods should *not* be initiated prior to 1 month postpartum for the breastfeeding woman?

a. Depot medroxyprogesterone acetate (DMPA) injection
b. Combination oral contraceptives
c. Etonogestrel implant (Implanon)
d. Progestin-only pills

99. The woman with postpartum thyroid dysfunction:

a. Almost always starts with symptoms of hyperthyroidism
b. May present initially with hypothyroidism changing to hyperthyroidism
c. May present with symptoms similar to postpartum depression
d. Rarely progresses to permanent hypothyroidism

100. When counseling the breast feeding mother concerning infant nutrition, she should be told that:

a. Iron fortified cereal or liquid iron should be started at about 3 months of age.
b. The iron in human milk is absorbed better by the infant than is iron in formula.

c. The breastfed infant does not need any vitamin or mineral supplements in the first 6 months.
d. Vitamin D and fluoride supplementation are recommended starting at 2 months.

101. All of the following drugs have been shown to have teratogenic effects except:

a. Anticonvulsants
b. Combination oral contraceptives
c. Isotretinoin
d. Oral anticoagulants

102. A 35-week-gestation G1 P0 tells you her friend's baby had jaundice and had to stay in the hospital for several days after birth. She asks what causes jaundice and could it happen after she takes her baby home. An appropriate response would be:

a. Jaundice that occurs after 24 hours is usually not an indicator of a serious problem.
b. Jaundice in the first 24 hours is an indicator of acute infection with hepatitis.
c. If the infant develops jaundice after discharge they will be readmitted for 24–48 hours of observation.
d. Because jaundice is caused by blood incompatibilities, she does not have to worry about this happening.

103. Which of the following statements concerning sudden infant death syndrome (SIDS) is correct?

a. Keeping the infant in the parent's bed during the night for the first 3 months may decrease the incidence of SIDS.
b. The occurrence of SIDS is rare in the first month of life and peaks between 2 and 3 months.
c. The risk for SIDS can be reduced by being sure the infant sleeps on a soft surface and is kept well covered.

d. There is no relationship between either gender or race and the incidence of SIDS.

104. A 21-year-old woman delivered her first baby 5 weeks ago. She had a normal spontaneous delivery. Her postpartum course has been unremarkable. She has been breastfeeding her infant on demand since birth and has had some problems with cracked nipples, but otherwise is satisfied with how well it is going. She calls the office today with the complaint of a headache, flu-like symptoms, tenderness of her right breast, and a temperature of 103°F. Management should include:

a. Washing the nipples with water only and applying a topical antifungal medication
b. Taking a mild analgesic, increasing fluids, and stopping breastfeeding for 24 hours
c. Admitting her to the hospital for 24 hours of IV antibiotics
d. Initiating antibiotics and advising her to take extra fluids and to nurse frequently

105. During childbirth preparation class a mother asks about the benefits and risks of epidural anesthesia. An appropriate response would include telling her that:

a. Small amounts of anesthetic are absorbed into the bloodstream so there is a risk for fetal hypotension.
b. Maternal hypotension is a possible complication and this may lead to fetal bradycardia.
c. Studies have shown that the use of epidural anesthesia often leads to a faster progression of labor.
d. Prior to epidural anesthesia a catheter is inserted in the bladder to prevent urinary retention.

106. Which of the following statements concerning postpartum depression is true?

a. The DSM-IV allows the specifier of "postpartum" to be used with depression if it occurs within the first 4 weeks postpartum.
b. Data indicate the cause of postpartum depression is related to psychosocial factors rather than hormonal changes.
c. The breastfeeding woman with postpartum depression should avoid the use of antidepressants.
d. If untreated, postpartum depression leads to psychosis in 2–3% of women.

107. Which of the following statements is *most* true regarding attachment and bonding between parents and babies?

a. The presence of extended family at the time of birth has been shown to be a strong factor in establishing a strong bond between infant and mother.
b. The attachment process occurs both prenatally and postpartum.
c. Allowing the mother to rest until the newborn is in the alert phase at about 2–3 hours after delivery facilitates bonding.
d. Mothers from virtually all cultures go through the same attachment and bonding activities.

108. In childbirth class you are discussing options for pain relief in labor. A couple asks about a pudendal block. You tell them this is a technique of injecting:

a. Local anesthetic into the subcutaneous tissue of the perineum to numb the area prior to episiotomy
b. An anesthetic into the caudal space in the spine to cause a numbing of the perineal area
c. An anesthetic transvaginally just prior to birth to numb the perineum and lower vagina
d. Regional anesthetic into the epidural space to provide relief from the pain of contractions

◘ ANSWERS AND RATIONALE

1.   **(a)** Elevated progesterone levels cause smooth muscle relaxation resulting in decreased peristalsis. This contributes to the common complaint of constipation during pregnancy (Lowdermilk & Perry, p. 349).

2.   **(c)** A prepregnant weight of 130 lbs. for a woman who is 5′ 6″ would be considered within normal limits (body mass index [BMI] 18.5–24.9). Recommended weight gain for the woman of normal weight is 25 to 35 lbs. A woman who is underweight (BMI less than 18.5) should gain 28 to 40 pounds, and a woman who is obese (BMI 30 or greater) should gain 11 to 20 lbs. (Institute of Medicine, p. 254).

3.   **(b)** The expected level of the fundus at 12 weeks is the symphysis pubis, at 16 weeks half way between the symphysis pubis and umbilicus, and at 20 weeks at or just below the umbilicus (Seidel et al., p. 617).

4.   **(b)** Heartburn is a common discomfort in the late second and third trimesters. Relaxation of the cardiac sphincter and decreased gastrointestinal motility contribute to heartburn. In addition, there is less room for the stomach to expand due to the increasing size of the uterus. Small, frequent meals may help to prevent heartburn by preventing overload of the stomach. Beverages should be avoided during meals as they tend to inhibit gastric juices. Lying down immediately after eating increases the likelihood for gastric reflux. Low sodium antacids may be used (Lowdermilk & Perry, p. 349; Tharpe & Farley, pp. 56–58).

5.   **(a)** Presumptive indicators of pregnancy are physiologic changes the woman experiences that suggest to her that she may be pregnant but that may be caused by other conditions. Probable indicators of pregnancy are detected by an examiner and relate mainly to physical changes in the uterus. Positive indicators are those directly attributable to the fetus as detected by an examiner such as the palpation of fetal movement, fetal heartbeat distinct from that of the mother, and viewing the fetus on ultrasound (Lowdermilk & Perry, p. 381).

6.   **(c)** Increases in both blood volume and cardiac output during pregnancy may cause some auscultatory changes. After 20 weeks, both components of the first heart sound become louder and there is an exaggerated splitting due to the increased circulating blood volume. There may also be audible splitting of S2, and S3 may be heard, as well as low-grade systolic and diastolic murmurs (Lowdermilk & Perry, p. 341).

7.   **(d)** G6 T3 P1 A1 L2. Gravida is any pregnancy, regardless of duration, including the present pregnancy. Term is delivery between the beginning of week 38 of gestation and the end of week 42 of gestation. Preterm is delivery after 20 weeks' gestation but before completion of 37 weeks' gestation. Spontaneous abortion refers to expulsion of the fetus prior to viability. Stillbirth refers to an infant born dead after 20 weeks' gestation. A stillbirth at 34 weeks' gestation would be considered a premature birth (Lowdermilk & Perry, p. 333).

8.   **(d)** hCG is produced by the trophoblast, and can be detected in the maternal serum by 8 to 10 days after conception, shortly after implantation (Lowdermilk & Perry, p. 319).

9.   **(a)** TSH levels remain within the normal, nonpregnant range during pregnancy. There is an estrogen induced increase in TBG. The increase in TBG results in an increase in total T_4 and T_3 levels. Concentrations of active thyroid hormones (free T_4 and T_3) do not

change during pregnancy (Lowder-milk & Perry, p. 350).

10. **(d)** Using Naegele's rule, one takes the first day of the last menstrual period, adds 7 days and then sub-tracts 3 months to get an EDD. 11/20 plus seven days = 11/27, minus three months = 8/27 (Lowdermilk & Perry, p. 381).

11. **(b)** The pregnant woman with a positive PPD test should have a chest radiograph preferably after the first trimester. An abdominal shield should be used to protect the fetus from radiation. Treatment regimens are determined by the results of the chest radiograph and by timing of serocon-version if known. If the chest radio-graph is negative for active TB but the pregnant woman is determined to be a recent converter, positive through exposure to active disease, or is HIV positive, treatment should still be initiated as active disease risk is high (Gibbs et al., pp. 292–293).

12. **(d)** The CDC recommends universal screening of pregnant women for HIV as part of routine early prenatal tests with option to decline (opt-out testing). Repeat testing in the third trimester should be considered if the woman has elevated risk factors for HIV infection (Branson et al., pp. 2–4).

13. **(d)** Chloasma, or the "mask of preg-nancy," is an irregular brownish dis-coloration of the forehead, cheeks, and nose. It is believed to be the result of the melanocyte stimulating effect of estrogen and progesterone. This discoloration usually fades and disappears after pregnancy has ended (Lowdermilk & Perry, p. 346).

14. **(a)** hPL stimulates growth of the breasts and has lactogenic properties in addition to having a number of metabolic effects (Lowdermilk & Perry, p. 320).

15. **(c)** Softening of the uterine isthmus (Hegar's sign) is evident at about 6 weeks' gestation. Braxton Hicks con-tractions may start as early as 6 weeks' gestation, but are not palpable until the second trimester. As the uterus be-comes an abdominal organ it rotates slightly to the right (dextrorotation). The uterus is palpable at the symphy-sis pubis at 12 weeks' gestation (Low-dermilk & Perry, pp. 336–337).

16. **(d)** Glomerular filtration rate and renal plasma flow increase early in pregnancy. Creatinine levels decrease. Tubular reabsorption of sodium in-creases. Reabsorption of glucose is impaired so glucosuria may occur during pregnancy. The possibility of gestational diabetes must, however, be kept in mind when glucose is per-sistently present in the urine (Lowder-milk & Perry, pp. 344–346).

17. **(b)** Hemodynamic changes that occur during pregnancy include increased cardiac output, heart rate, and blood volume. There is a slight decrease in systolic and diastolic blood pressure in the second trimester, with return to prepregnancy levels late in the third trimester. Red blood cell mass in-creases, although the rapid expansion of blood volume causes a hemodilu-tion with expected decreases in hemo-globin and hematocrit. White blood cell production increases in the second and third trimesters (Lowdermilk & Perry, pp. 340–344).

18. **(c)** A clean catch urine sample show-ing the presence of 50,000 pathogenic bacteria of the same species per mL with no urinary tract infection symp-toms is indicative of asymptomatic bacteriuria. Because untreated asymp-tomatic bacteriuria is associated with pyelonephritis, preterm labor, and low birth weight, it should be treated with the appropriate antibiotic. A repeat urine culture after treat-ment is needed (Tharpe & Farley, pp. 106–109).

19. **(c)** Leg cramps are a common discomfort in the third trimester of pregnancy. The exact cause is unknown. Changes in calcium and phosphorus metabolism and pressure from the enlarging uterus on pelvic nerves and blood vessels are possible causes. Dorsiflexing the foot is helpful as this stretches the calf muscle. Walking promotes circulation and stretches the calf muscles as long as high heeled shoes are avoided. Dietary increase in magnesium may be considered as most women have inadequate intake of this mineral that aids in muscle relaxation. (Tharpe & Farley, pp. 61–62).

20. **(c)** Current recommendations are that women should take 0.4 mg of folic acid daily both before conception and during the first trimester to help prevent neural tube defects. Women with a history of a previous pregnancy with a neural tube defect should begin taking 4 mg of folic acid daily for the month prior to conception and during the first trimester (Gabbe et al., p. 117).

21. **(c)** The blastocyst develops into the embryo, amnion, and yolk sac membrane (Lowdermilk & Perry, pp. 315–318).

22. **(b)** The most highly sensitive time for a teratogenic effect on the heart is between weeks 3 and 8. The entire embryonic period is a critical time for teratogenesis that may be lethal or cause major congenital malformations (Lowdermilk & Perry, p. 317).

23. **(b)** The corpus luteum is responsible for secreting estrogen and progesterone to maintain early pregnancy. It remains functional during the first few months of pregnancy until the placenta takes over this function (Lowdermilk & Perry, pp. 319–320).

24. **(c)** A woman who is currently pregnant and has had two miscarriages (has not completed a pregnancy with fetus or fetuses who have reached 20 weeks' gestation) is a nullipara and a multigravida (Lowdermilk & Perry, p. 333).

25. **(c)** There is no evidence of fetal risk from toxoid vaccines such as the tetanus vaccine or from tetanus immune globulin. Recommendations are to administer a booster if more than 5 years have elapsed since the last dose with this type of wound (CDC, 2010, pp. 2–3).

26. **(c)** Most (95%) reproductive age women are immune to varicella. When immunity of the pregnant woman is not certain, varicella serology (IgG antibody) should be obtained. Positive IgG antibody confirms immunity. If IgG antibody is absent, she should receive VZIG within 4 days of exposure (Gibbs et al., pp. 343–345).

27. **(c)** Amniocentesis is used in prenatal diagnosis of genetic disorders and congenital anomalies, assessment of fetal lung maturity, and diagnosis of fetal hemolytic disease (Lowdermilk & Perry, pp. 774–775).

28. **(c)** The results of a nonstress test are considered reassuring when there is a minimum of two or more accelerations in the fetal heart rate of 15 or more beats for 15 or more seconds in a 20-minute period (Lowdermilk & Perry, p. 779).

29. **(d)** Vena cava syndrome or supine hypotension occurs when the pregnant woman lies in a supine position, because of the weight of the uterus and fetus on the inferior vena cava. The woman may feel dizzy, lightheaded and may even have syncope. Symptoms can be alleviated by having the woman turn on her side (Lowdermilk & Perry, p. 398).

30. **(d)** A biophysical profile (BPP) of 6 out of 10 with a normal amniotic fluid volume is considered to be equivocal and suspicious for chronic asphyxia. Delivery is indicated if the fetus is 36 weeks' gestation with tests indicating lung maturity. If the lungs are not mature, repeat testing in 4–6 hours. If oligohydramnios is present, delivery is indicated (Gabbe et al., p. 283).

31. **(b)** There are several different counting methods. In the Count-to-Ten method, the woman starts counting movements in the morning and records the time of day when she has perceived 10 movements. If there are fewer than 10 movements in 12 hours, or if takes longer each day to reach 10 movements, the woman should contact her healthcare provider for further evaluation. Periods of active movement last about 40 minutes and quiet periods about 20 minutes. Fetal activity does not necessarily increase after a meal. Fetal activity does not normally decrease as the woman nears term. There is a clearly established relationship between decreased fetal activity and fetal distress (Gabbe et al., pp. 272–274; Lowdermilk & Perry, p. 767).

32. **(a)** Bishop's scoring is done to evaluate cervical readiness for induction. The five factors evaluated include dilatation, effacement, station, cervix consistency, and cervix position (Lowdermilk & Perry, p. 948).

33. **(d)** The monitor strip shows late decelerations. This type of deceleration is most commonly seen with uteroplacental insufficiency. Early decelerations may be seen with head compression and are usually benign. Variable decelerations are seen with cord compression (Lowdermilk & Perry, pp. 504–509).

34. **(d)** Positioning a woman on her left side will increase the blood flow to the uterus. Administering oxygen at 8 to 10 liters/min will increase the amount available to the fetus between contractions. Hydration should be maintained with an IV and if oxytocin is being administered, it should be discontinued (Lowdermilk & Perry, pp. 508–509).

35. **(d)** A negative contraction stress test (CST) indicates there were no late decelerations with adequate uterine contractions (3 in 10 minutes). A negative CST has consistently been associated with good fetal outcome. It is considered to be predictive for 7 days, so weekly retesting is appropriate when using the CST to screen for uteroplacental insufficiency (Gibbs et al., p. 160; Lowdermilk & Perry, pp. 779–781).

36. **(c)** The vaginal examination findings of 50%, 3 cm, –1 describe a cervix that is 50% effaced, 3 cm dilated, and fetal presenting part that is 1 cm (–1 station) above the ischial spines. The fetal presenting part is considered floating when it is at –5 station (Lowdermilk & Perry, pp. 450–452, 455–456).

37. **(b)** Implantation occurs between days 7 and 9 after fertilization. An abortion is classified as inevitable when there is cervical dilatation or rupture of membranes. With an incomplete abortion the internal os will be dilated slightly and bleeding is often profuse. With an ectopic pregnancy the uterus may be slightly enlarged. This client's symptoms and physical examination findings may be indicative of either a threatened abortion or an ectopic pregnancy (Gibbs et al., pp. 62, 74; Lowdermilk & Perry, pp. 806–807, 811–812).

38. **(a)** Nonmeat foods that are high in iron include iron fortified cereals, soybeans, roasted pumpkin and squash seeds, white beans, lentils, and black

strap molasses (Tharpe & Farley, p. 437).

39. **(b)** CDC treatment guidelines state that podophyllin, podofilox, and imiquimod should not be used during pregnancy. Treatment during pregnancy with trichloroacetic acid or cryotherapy may be considered as genital warts often proliferate and become friable during pregnancy (CDC, 2010, p. 66).

40. **(d)** A sterile speculum examination may be done to assess for rupture of membranes along with inspection for cord prolapse, assessment of cervical dilatation and effacement, and to obtain cultures. The pH of amniotic fluid is 7.1 to 7.3. Other factors that can cause an alkaline pH include blood, semen, and bacterial vaginosis or trichomoniasis (ACOG, 2007, pp. 966–967).

41. **(a)** For an infant to have sickle cell disease, both parents must have the trait and the child must inherit the trait from both parents. With an autosomal recessive trait, this is a one in four chance (Lowdermilk & Perry, p. 63).

42. **(a)** Prenatal screening for Group B streptococcus (GBS) is recommended for all pregnant women at 35 to 37 weeks' gestation. The specimen for culture should be obtained from the lower vagina (vaginal introitus) and rectum (through the anal sphincter). Women with positive culture should receive antibiotic prophylaxis during labor (Gibbs et al., pp. 340–343).

43. **(a)** Information concerning chromosomal status and DNA patterns can be obtained through chorionic villi sampling (CVS). Information that requires amniotic fluid, such as an alpha-fetoprotein (AFP) to detect neural tube abnormalities, cannot be obtained. Studies concerning limb reduction defects related to CVS indicate that the greatest risk is associated with the procedure performed at less than 10 weeks' gestation. Pregnancy loss rates with CVS have been shown to be no different from loss rates after amniocentesis when the healthcare provider is experienced in performing the procedure (Gibbs et al., pp. 117–119).

44. **(c)** Chronic hypertension is considered to be one of the many risk factors for intrauterine growth retardation (IUGR). Other risk factors include poor maternal nutrition, smoking, diabetes, substance abuse, short interpregnancy interval, multiple gestation, and abnormalities of the placenta (Gibbs et al., pp. 205–206; Lowdermilk & Perry, p. 765).

45. **(c)** When excessive fetomaternal bleeding is a concern with an Rh negative client, a Kliehauer-Betke test can be used to determine the volume of fetal red blood cells in the maternal circulation. The appropriate dose of Rh immune globulin to be given can be calculated according to the results of this test (Lowdermilk & Perry, p. 603).

46. **(c)** Methotrexate is a folic acid antagonist that interferes with DNA synthesis and cell multiplication (Gibbs et al., p. 77).

47. **(b)** Because methotrexate is a folic acid antagonist, the client should avoid any supplements containing folic acid during treatment (Lowdermilk & Perry, p. 813).

48. **(d)** Most women can continue to exercise safely during pregnancy with some precautions. Running is an acceptable form of exercise during pregnancy if the woman is already in a regular running program and not having any problems with the pregnancy. Precautions include limiting exercise

sessions to no more than 60 minutes to reduce any risk of fetal hyperthermia, stopping exercise if she feels fatigued, keeping heart rate at about 65 to 70% of maximal heart rate, not exercising in hot weather, and attending to hydration. She should also exercise 3 or 4 times a week as layoffs followed by quick returns increase the risk for injury. Caloric intake needed is directly influenced by a woman's activity level. She must monitor her weight gain to assure that she is getting adequate calories (Gibbs et al., 16–17).

49. **(d)** Chronic hypertension is a major risk factor for placental abruption. Maternal age older than 35 is also a risk factor. Signs and symptoms of placental abruption may include bleeding (although it may be concealed), back pain, colicky abdominal pain, and increased uterine tone between contractions. Depending on the degree of separation there may be abnormalities in fetal heart rate pattern, a decrease or absence of fetal activity, and signs of maternal shock (Gibbs et al., pp. 392–394; Lowdermilk & Perry, pp. 819–820).

50. **(d)** Ultrasound provides for evaluation of the fetus, placenta, and uterus. Continuous fetal monitoring is designed to observe for signs of decreased long-term variability indicating fetal stress, and for signs of uterine tetany and/or late decelerations. Since placental abruption frequently stimulates the clotting cascade resulting in DIC, coagulation studies including fibrinogen, platelet count, PT, and PTT should be measured (Gibbs et al., pp. 395–397; Lowdermilk & Perry, pp. 821–822).

51. **(a)** Risk factors for placental abruption include but are not limited to hypertension, high parity, preterm rupture of membranes with chorioamnionitis, smoking, cocaine use, blunt abdominal trauma, sudden decompression of the uterus (amniocentesis), incorrectly applied seat belt and thrombophilias. (Gibbs et al., pp. 393–394).

52. **(c)** HELLP stands for hemolysis, elevated liver enzymes, and low platelets. These are the physiologic abnormalities that may be seen with progressive preeclampsia (Lowdermilk & Perry, p. 788).

53. **(c)** Chronic hypertension is defined as BP 140/90 or greater diagnosed prior to pregnancy, prior to 20 weeks' gestation, or that persists after 12 weeks postpartum. Preeclampsia is defined as BP 140/90 or greater occurring after 20 weeks' gestation accompanied by proteinuria. Preeclampsia superimposed on chronic hypertension is defined as meeting the criteria for chronic hypertension with new onset of proteinuria after 20 weeks' gestation (Gibbs et al., pp. 258–259).

54. **(d)** Risk factors for asymptomatic bacteriuria in pregnancy include a history of urinary tract infections, diabetes, and sickle cell trait/disease. Untreated asymptomatic bacteriuria is associated with pyelonephritis, preterm delivery, and low birth weight (Tharpe & Farley, p. 106).

55. **(a)** In late pregnancy there is accelerated growth of the fetus and an increased need for glucose by the fetoplacental unit; increase in several diabetogenic hormones including human placental lactogen, cortisol, progesterone, and estrogens; and increasing insulin resistance in both the periphery (muscle) and hepatic levels. In a normal pregnancy the pancreas is able to produce sufficient insulin to compensate for insulin resistance and to maintain euglycemia (Gibbs et al., pp. 246–247; Lowdermilk & Perry, p. 839).

56. **(c)** ACOG recommendations are that either universal or selective screening for gestational diabetes mellitus (GDM) be performed at 24 to 28 weeks of gestation. Women who are low risk are the only ones who do not need to be screened. Low risk is defined as having all of the following characteristics: member of ethnic group with low prevalence of GDM, no known diabetes in first degree relatives, age younger than 25 years, normal prepregnancy weight, no history of abnormal glucose metabolism, and no history of poor obstetric outcome (Gabbe et al., pp. 992–993).

57. **(c)** The diagnosis of gestational diabetes is made when any two of the following glucose values on plasma samples are met or exceeded: Fasting—105 mg, 1 hour—190 mg, 2 hour—165 mg, 3 hour—145 mg (Gabbe et al., p. 994).

58. **(a)** The glycosylated hemoglobin (Hgb A_{1c}) provides an accurate long-term index of the client's average blood glucose over the previous 8 to 12 weeks. This would be useful in helping the client to obtain strict control of her glucose levels prior to pregnancy. Strict diabetes control prior to pregnancy and early in pregnancy may reduce the risk for congenital anomalies that are more common with maternal diabetes. It is unlikely that she will be switched to an oral hypoglycemic during her pregnancy if she is currently using insulin. Glyburide has been shown to be a safe and effective alternative to insulin for women with GDM. The need for insulin frequently decreases in the first trimester and then begins to rise in the second trimester. Fetal macrosomia results when there are high levels of maternal glucose. Strict glucose control during pregnancy may reduce this risk (Gabbe et al., p. 1001; Gibbs et al., pp. 249–250, 252).

59. **(b)** The ultimate goal of asthma therapy during pregnancy is to maintain optimal fetal oxygenation by preventing maternal hypoxic events. Budesonide is the preferred inhaled corticosteroid for use during pregnancy. Inhaled albuterol is the recommended rescue therapy during pregnancy. Both of these medications may be used during labor and delivery and while breastfeeding. Asthma is usually quiescent during labor but ongoing assessment of untoward signs or symptoms as well as peak expiratory flow rate evaluation is important (ACOG, 2008, pp. 1014–1017; Gabbe et al., pp. 949–955).

60. **(b)** Aspirin decreases platelet aggregation, which can increase the risk of bleeding before and during delivery. There is also some risk of premature closure of the fetal ductus arteriosis with the prostoglandin synthetase inhibitors such as aspirin, ibuprofen, and naproxen. Acetaminophen use does not have these potential adverse effects and is preferred when a mild analgesic or antipyretic is indicated. Nonmedication remedies should be considered for first line relief to include humidifiers, rest, and fluids. If a decongestant is needed, a nasal spray is preferred to an oral decongestant as topical administration results in a lower dose to the fetus (Gabbe et al., pp. 196–197, 199).

61. **(c)** The indirect Coombs test (antibody screen) determines if the mother has any antibodies to Rh positive blood. The test is routinely done for Rh negative women at their initial visit and at 27 to 28 weeks. If the test is positive it indicates that the mother has already been sensitized; RhoGAM is used to prevent sensitization but does not reverse preexisting sensitization. If the baby is Rh negative, RhoGAM is not needed. Therefore it is the mother with a negative indirect Coombs and an Rh positive baby who

will benefit from receiving RhoGAM after delivery (Gibbs et al., p. 319; Lowdermilk & Perry, pp. 603–604).

62. **(a)** Kell refers to the K or K1 antigen of the Kell blood group system. About 0.2% of pregnant women are positive for anti-Kell with nearly all cases of isoimmunization occurring as a result of a Kell-incompatible transfusion. Kell isoimmunization can result in erythroblastosis fetalis. RhoGAM is not effective in preventing Kell isoimmunization (Gabbe et al., pp. 829–830).

63. **(c)** ABO incompatibility is a common cause of hemolytic disease in the newborn. However, it rarely results in severe hemolytic disease, with less than 1% requiring exchange transfusions. It usually manifests itself as mild to moderate hyperbilirubinemia during the first 24 to 48 hours of life. ABO incompatibility occurs when the mother's blood type is O and the infant's blood type is A or B (Gibbs et al., p. 326; Lowdermilk & Perry, p. 1027).

64. **(b)** Spectrophotometric analysis of amniotic fluid bilirubin levels correlate with the severity of fetal hemolysis in Rh isoimmunization. The Liley graph (optical density graph) is used to plot the serial measurement of bilirubin in the amniotic fluid as determined by spectrophotometry. The results on the graph are used to place the fetus in zones representing unaffected to severely affected. The graph is used to help clinicians in making decisions about the timing of delivery. Serial amniocentesis has been replaced in some centers with fetal middle cerebral artery (MCA) Doppler measurement to assess for fetal anemia (Gabbe et al., pp. 822–824; Gibbs et al., pp. 321–322).

65. **(b)** MSAFP is designed as a screening test to be performed between 15 and 22 weeks' gestation. Results are most accurate when performed between 16 and 18 weeks. The most common reason for a false positive is incorrect dates. Undiagnosed multiple gestation may also cause a false positive. If the results come back abnormal, ultrasound should be scheduled. The ultrasound will help in determining an accurate gestational date or presence of multiple gestations (Gabbe et al., 168–169; Gibbs et al., pp. 113–114).

66. **(b)** FAS (fetal alcohol syndrome) is now believed to be the number one preventable birth defect. Down syndrome and some neural tube defects may be genetically based, and IUGR is not a birth defect (Lowdermilk & Perry, pp. 1013–1014).

67. **(c)** Serial cervical and vaginal cultures have not been shown to be predictive for newborn infection. Routine Cesarean delivery is not recommended. Cesarean delivery is recommended if a lesion or prodromal symptoms are present at onset of labor. Data indicate a significant reduction in recurrences at time of delivery, reduction of C-sections, and decrease in viral detection at delivery with use of suppressive therapy starting at 36 weeks in women with recurrent herpes (ACOG, 2007, pp. 980–982).

68. **(b)** Asymmetric intrauterine growth restriction is most likely to occur when there is a uteroplacental insufficiency starting in later pregnancy after the growth in number of cells is complete. Growth of the fetus in the third trimester is characterized by growth in the size of existing cells (hypertrophy) rather than growth in number of cells (hyperplasia). With asymmetric intrauterine growth restriction there is a reduction in hepatic glucose stores that reduces liver size and results in an increase in head circumference to abdominal circumference. There is also a redistribution of fetal blood flow to the vital organs including the heart

and brain. There is normal growth of the brain and head compared with slower growth in abdomen and extremities (Gibbs et al., p. 203).

69. **(c)** TORCH is an acronym for a variety of infections that may cause harm to the fetus during pregnancy. It stands for Toxoplasmosis, Other infections (e.g., hepatitis, varicella), Rubella, Cytomegalovirus (CMV) and Herpes simplex. The organisms causing these infections are capable of crossing the placenta (Lowdermilk & Perry, p. 199).

70. **(c)** About 65% of pregnant women are immune to fifth disease (human parvovirus). Susceptible women have a 50% risk of infection following exposure. Infection occurs in about 33% of fetuses when maternal infection occurs. Fetal death is approximately 11% when infection occurs during the first half of pregnancy and is rare when infection occurs after 20 weeks' gestation. Fetal hydrops may occur. (Gabbe et al., pp. 1213–1215).

71. **(b)** Polyhydramnios is associated with diabetes, GI tract anomalies, neural tube defects, Rh isoimmunization, and multiple gestations. Potential complications with polyhydramnios include preterm labor, placental abruption, prolapsed cord with rupture of membranes, and postpartum hemorrhage because of uterine overdistention (Gabbe et al., p. 840).

72. **(c)** Oligohydramnios is associated with major fetal renal malformations. It may also be found with premature rupture of membranes, postterm pregnancy, and with IUGR that is secondary to placental insufficiency (Gabbe et al., p. 839; Lowdermilk & Perry, p. 141).

73. **(b)** A definitive diagnosis of antiphospholipid syndrome is made when at least one of the clinical and one of the laboratory criteria are met. The clinical criteria are vascular thrombosis (one or more episodes confirmed by imaging or Doppler studies without significant inflammation of vessel wall) and pregnancy morbidity (one or more unexplained deaths of normal fetus after the 10th week of gestation; OR one or more premature births of normal neonate at or before the 34th week of gestation because of severe preeclampsia or severe placental insufficiency; OR three or more consecutive spontaneous abortions prior to the 10th week of gestation). The laboratory criteria are presence of anticardiolipin antibody of IgG and/or IgM isotope on at least two or more occasions at least 6 weeks apart, and presence of lupus anticoagulant on two or more occasions at least 6 weeks apart (Gabbe et al., p. 1088).

74. **(a)** Contraction frequency is timed from the beginning of one contraction to the beginning of the next contraction (Lowdermilk & Perry, p. 455).

75. **(c)** Second degree lacerations include the vaginal mucosa, posterior fourchette, perineal skin, and perineal muscles. There is no extension into the external anal sphincter (Lowdermilk & Perry, p. 565).

76. **(c)** The first stage of labor is defined as beginning with true labor contractions, which cause progressive cervical dilatation and ending with the cervix being completely dilated (Lowdermilk & Perry, p. 519).

77. **(a)** ACOG recommendations are that the FHR should be auscultated at least every 30 minutes just after a contraction in the active phase of the first stage of labor, and at least every 15 minutes during the second stage of labor in someone with no risk factors (Lowdermilk & Perry, p. 499).

78. **(d)** The seven cardinal movements in the normal mechanism of labor that

occur in vertex position are engagement, descent, flexion, internal rotation, extension, external rotation or restitution, and birth by expulsion (Lowdermilk & Perry, pp. 460–463).

79. **(b)** VBAC contraindications include circumstances that would place the woman at high risk for uterine rupture. A trial of labor should not be attempted if (1) there was a prior classical or T-shaped uterine incision; (2) there was a previous uterine rupture; (3) there is a medical or obstetric complication precluding vaginal delivery; or (4) if there is not the capability to perform an immediate emergency C-section if needed. Given this client's history of "a little extra cut" on the uterine incision, she most likely had a classical or T-shaped incision (Gabbe et al., pp. 492–493, 502).

80. **(b)** Fetal activity is extremely sensitive to decreases in fetal oxygenation. A decrease or absence of fetal movement requires further assessment with a nonstress test and other tests as indicated by findings (Gabbe et al., pp. 273–275).

81. **(b)** The woman/couple should be encouraged to make as many choices as possible about medical care including the timing of delivery. Most women choose to be delivered as soon as possible; however, it is acceptable to wait until spontaneous labor begins (usually within 2 to 3 weeks of fetal death). Maternal coagulopathy and intrauterine infection are rare. It is reasonable to monitor a woman with serial assessment of temperature, abdominal pain, malodorous vaginal discharge, bleeding, and labor. The benefit of serial determination of WBC count and coagulation status is uncertain (Gibbs et al., p. 425).

82. **(c)** Complications associated with postterm pregnancy include shoulder dystocia and fetal injury related to macrosomia, increased chance of operative delivery, meconium aspiration, placental insufficiency, and oligohydramnios (Gibbs et al., p. 181).

83. **(c)** Magnesium sulfate ($MgSO_4$) acts as a CNS depressant. Its primary use with severe preeclampsia is seizure prevention. Because it secondarily relaxes smooth muscle, it may also reduce blood pressure and decrease the frequency and intensity of contractions (Gabbe et al., p. 887; Lowdermilk & Perry, pp. 796–798).

84. **(d)** Early symptoms of $MgSO_4$ toxicity include nausea, warmth, and flushing. Signs of $MgSO_4$ toxicity include depression or absence of reflexes, oliguria, confusion, and respiratory depression (Lowdermilk & Perry, p. 798).

85. **(b)** The antidote for $MgSO_4$ toxicity is calcium gluconate (Lowdermilk & Perry, p. 798).

86. **(a)** Hydatidiform moles occur most frequently in women in their early teens and in older women, especially those older than 45 years. Signs and symptoms may include vaginal bleeding, hyperemesis gravidarum, gestational hypertension before 20 weeks' gestation, and uterus that is large for gestational dates. Fetal heart tones are absent. Vesicular tissue may be passed with vaginal bleeding. Ultrasound will show a characteristic mixed echogenic "snowstorm" image filling the uterus. (Gibbs et al, pp. 1071–1074; Lowdermilk & Perry, 814–815).

87. **(d)** Oxytocin is produced in the posterior pituitary gland and is responsible for the let-down reflex. This hormone also stimulates uterine contractions that promote uterine involution. Oxytocin is released in response to stimulation of the nipple by the suckling infant. It may also be released in response to sights, sounds, or odors the

mother associates with her baby and in response to orgasm (Lowdermilk & Perry, p. 717).

88. **(d)** The most common presentation for a twin gestation is a large for dates uterus and possibly exaggerated symptoms of pregnancy. A woman may also complain of early or excessive fetal movement, and two fetal heart tones may be auscultated. Another reason for excessive nausea and vomiting and increased fundal height may be a hydatidiform mole. The distinction would be uterine bleeding by the 12th week and no fetal heart tones. The initial step in this situation would be to obtain an ultrasound. Accurate gestational dating and determination of multiple gestation are important prior to an MSAFP (Gabbe et al., pp. 168, 735)

89. **(c)** Potential complications for the fetus in a multiple gestation pregnancy include preterm birth, SGA, IUGR, cord accidents, malpresentation, congenital anomalies, and twin to twin transfusion. For the mother, potential complications include PIH, placental abruption, preterm labor and postpartum hemorrhage (Gibbs, et al., pp. 223–230).

90. **(c)** Delivery of a girl and boy tells you they are dizygotic or fraternal twins. Dizygotic twins always have dichorionic-diamniotic placentas although they may be fused (Gabbe et al., pp. 736–737; Lowdermilk & Perry, p. 327).

91. **(c)** Sterile speculum examination should be performed to evaluate membrane status and to obtain cultures for group B streptococcus, chlamydia, and gonorrhea. Digital examination should only be performed after rupture of membranes has been ruled out. Transabdominal ultrasound may be useful in confirming gestational age, determining placental location, and determining presentation. A biophysical profile might be indicated if the nonstress test was nonreactive (Gabbe et al., p. 685).

92. **(b)** The specimen for the group B streptococcus culture should be obtained from the outer one third of the vagina and the rectum. The specimen for the fern pattern test should be obtained from fluid in the posterior vaginal fornix or from fluid coming out of the cervical os. The specimen for pH testing can be obtained from the blade of the speculum to obtain fluid from the posterior fornix. A specimen taken from the cervical os may produce a false positive color change as well as a false positive ferning pattern because cervical mucus may be alkaline. The specimen for the fibronectin assay should be obtained from the external cervical os and the posterior fornix (Gabbe et al., pp. 685, 717).

93. **(d)** Administration of corticosteroids to women between 24 and 34 weeks' gestation has been demonstrated to induce fetal lung maturity and to decrease the incidence of respiratory distress syndrome. Other preterm related morbidities that are reduced include intraventricular hemorrhage, patent ductus arteriosus, bronchopulmonary dysplasia, and necrotizing enterocolitis (Gabbe et al., p. 686).

94. **(a)** Terbutaline is a beta adrenergic agonist. It stimulates the beta receptors resulting in smooth muscle relaxation. Pulmonary edema is the most serious complication with the use of terbutaline. Other side-effects include tachycardia, hypotension, hyperglycemia, hypokalemia, and jitteriness (Gabbe et al., pp. 691–692).

95. **(a)** Lochia rubra is bright red and is seen for the first 2 to 3 days postpartum. Immediately after delivery the vagina appears stretched and there may be some erythema and edema at

the introitus. The fundus is about 2 cm below the umbilicus right after delivery and then may rise to about 1 cm above the umbilicus within 12 hours postpartum. If the fundus remains above the umbilicus, consider the possibility of filling of the uterus with blood clots or displacement by a distended bladder (Lowdermilk & Perry, pp. 576–579).

96. **(b)** The white cell count may be elevated to between 20,000 to 25,000 mm³ the first several days postpartum. A temperature up to 100.4°F may occur in the first 24 hours postpartum as a result of the exertion and dehydration of labor (Lowdermilk & Perry, pp. 582–583).

97. **(d)** For women who choose not to breast feed, suppression of lactation may be enhanced by wearing a supportive, well fitting brassiere continuously for the first 5 to 7 days postpartum, removing the bra only for showering. When showering, she should avoid letting warm water directly hit her breasts as this has a stimulating effect. Warm compresses would also have a stimulating effect. Ice packs and mild analgesics may be used if needed for discomfort. Although bromocriptine was used in the past for lactation suppression, it is no longer recommended due to potential adverse reactions (Gabbe et al., pp. 576–577; Lowdermilk & Perry, p. 582).

98. **(b)** US Medical Eligibility Criteria for Contraceptive Use include DMPA, progestin-only pills, and etonogestrel implant (Implanon) for breastfeeding women less than 1 month postpartum as methods for which the advantages generally outweigh the theoretical or proven risks (Category 2). Combination oral contraceptives use by breastfeeding women less than 1 month postpartum is considered Category 3 for which the theoretical or proven risks usually outweigh the advantages of using the method (CDC, Appendix A).

99. **(c)** The clinical course for postpartum thyroid dysfunction is variable. About one third will first have hyperthyroidism and then develop hypothyroidism, one third have hypothyroidism without preceding hyperthyroidism, and one third have hyperthyroidism that resolves without hypothyroidism. Although uncommon, the hypothyroidism may become permanent but usually resolves at least temporarily. About 50% of women with postpartum thyroid hypothyroidism will develop permanent hypothyroidism within 5 years. The woman with postpartum thyroid dysfunction may present with vague symptoms to include fatigue, tiredness, depression, palpitations, and irritability. It is necessary to evaluate for both thyroid dysfunction and postpartum depression (Gabbe et al., pp. 1030–1031).

100. **(b)** Supplementation of iron is not usually needed before the age of 6 months in the healthy breastfed infant. While the iron that is normally found in human milk may be at lower concentrations than that in prepared formulas, it is better absorbed by the infant. It is recommended that no fluoride supplement be given prior to 6 months of age. At 6 months of age, the infant may be given a fluoride supplement depending on the concentration of fluoride in the water supply. All breastfed infants should receive 200 IU of oral vitamin D drops daily beginning during the first 2 months and continuing until daily consumption of vitamin D fortified formula or milk is 500 mL (American Academy of Pediatrics, pp. 499–500).

101. **(b)** No association has been found between the use of combination oral contraceptives during pregnancy and fetal malformations. The risk for major fetal malformations when

the pregnant woman takes anticonvulsants is 5% compared with the general risk of 2–3%. Isotretinoin (Accutane) is known to be a significant human teratogen. Malformations occur in about 5% of fetuses when the mother takes warfarin (Coumadin) during early pregnancy (Gabbe et al., pp. 189–193).

102. **(a)** Physiologic jaundice occurs in about 50% of term infants and 80% of preterm infants. It typically occurs more than 24 hours after birth. It is more common in the breastfeeding infant but usually does not necessitate cessation of breastfeeding, with maximum bilirubin levels of 10–30 mg/dL that drop gradually over 3–12 weeks. Pathologic jaundice is usually first observed at less than 24 hours after birth, and there may be significant hyperbilirubinemia. The most common cause is hemolysis caused by fetomaternal blood incompatibilities or genetic disorders. Bilirubin overproduction may also be caused by polycythemia, increased enterohepatic circulation with gastrointestinal obstruction, sequestered blood (e.g., cephalohematoma, hemangiomas), or hepatic cell damage related to infection or drugs (Gabbe et al., pp. 545–546).

103. **(b)** The incidence of SIDS is rare during the first month of life, peaks in the second and third months and then decreases. There are consistently higher rates of SIDS in males and African-American, Native American, and Alaska Native children. The risk for SIDS is significantly reduced by keeping the baby supine, on a firm mattress with no extra pillows, and avoiding overheating while sleeping. While keeping the baby in the parent's bed at night is controversial, there is no data showing that it reduces the risks for SIDS, and in some studies an increased incidence of

SIDS has been demonstrated (American Academy of Pediatrics, 2005, pp. 1245–1248).

104. **(d)** Predisposing factors for mastitis include trauma to the breast (cracked nipples), primiparity, lactation, and stasis of human milk. Signs of mastitis include rapid elevation of temperature to 103° to 104°F, increased pulse rate, chills, malaise, headache, and an area on the breast that is red, tender, and hard. Treatment includes antibiotic therapy, rest, frequent breast feeding with emptying of the breasts to prevent stasis, and analgesics for pain and fever. Fungal mastitis is usually characterized by bilateral breast erythema and nipple tenderness. If mild it may be treated with topical antifungal medicine or if needed with systemic fluconazole. The infant may continue to breastfeed during treatment (Gabbe et al., p. 576).

105. **(b)** One of the most common sideeffects of epidural anesthesia is maternal hypotension with a resultant fetal bradycardia. Trace amounts of anesthetic are absorbed but there is no significant effect on the fetus. Loss of bladder sensation may occur leading to urinary retention. If this does occur, catheterization may be necessary during labor or the immediate postpartum. Although there is controversy regarding the effect on the progress of labor, some studies indicate that the use of epidural anesthesia may slow the progress of labor (Lowdermilk & Perry, pp. 485–488).

106. **(a)** The DSM-IV allows the designation of postpartum onset as a specifier for depression if it begins within 4 weeks postpartum, and the International Classification of Diseases permits the designation of postpartum depression if the disorder begins within the first 6 weeks postpartum. More research about the etiology and

effect of childbearing on psychiatric illness would be beneficial in establishing a consensus on the definition. Postpartum depression may last from months to years if unrecognized or untreated. It is likely that the etiology of postpartum depression is multifactoral, including genetics, hormonal changes, previous history of depression, physical environment, and social environment. Treatment measures include medication, individual or group psychotherapy, support groups, and assistance with childcare and other demands of daily living. Treatment with sertraline, paroxetine, and nortriptyline usually produce nonquantifiable levels in breastfed infants. Postpartum psychosis has an incidence of 1 to 2 per 1000 and usually is evident within 3 months postpartum (Lowdermilk & Perry, pp. 912–915; Gabbe et al., pp. 1255–1256).

107. **(b)** Maternal–infant attachment starts in the prenatal period, extends through labor/giving birth, into the early postpartum, and the initial caretaking time. The first 60 to 90 minutes after birth when the infant is in the alert stage allows for meaningful interaction between both parents and infant. Parents should be able to have time alone with the infant during this period if the infant's medical condition permits. Cultural background influences the mother's and father's behaviors during the postpartum period and should be considered when assessing maternal and paternal attachment (Gabbe et al., p. 557; Lowdermilk & Perry, p. 605).

108. **(c)** In a pudendal block, anesthetic is injected transvaginally into the pudendal nerve, which results in numbing of the perineum and outer vaginal area. It is not effective for labor pain but is used to numb the perineal area for delivery and/or repair (Gabbe et al., pp. 414–415; Lowdermilk & Perry, pp. 481–482).

◻ REFERENCES

American Academy of Pediatrics. (2005). Policy statement: Breastfeeding and the use of human milk. *Pediatrics, 115*(2), 496–506.

American Academy of Pediatrics Task Force on Sudden Infant Death Syndrome. (2005). The changing concept of sudden infant death syndrome: Diagnostic coding shifts, controversies regarding the sleeping environment and new variables to consider in reducing risk. *Pediatrics, 116*(5), 1245–1255.

American College of Obstetricians and Gynecologists (ACOG). (2007). Management of herpes in pregnancy. *Practice Bulletin No. 82.* Washington, DC: Author.

American College of Obstetricians and Gynecologists (ACOG). (2007). Premature rupture of membranes. *Practice Bulletin No. 80.* Washington, DC: Author.

American College of Obstetricians and Gynecologists (ACOG). (2008). Asthma in pregnancy. *Practice Bulletin No. 90.* Washington, DC: Author.

Branson, B., Handsfield, H., Lampe, M., et al. (2006). Revised recommendations for HIV testing of adults, adolescents, and pregnant women in healthcare settings. *Morbidity and Mortality Weekly Report, 55*(RR14).

Centers for Disease Control and Prevention (CDC). (2010). US medical eligibility criteria for contraceptive use, 2010. *Morbidity and Mortality Weekly Report, 59*(RR04).

Centers for Disease Control and Prevention (CDC). (2010). Quick guide: Recommended adult immunization schedule—US. 2010. *Morbidity and Mortality Weekly Report, 59*(1).

Centers for Disease Control and Prevention (CDC). (2006). Guidelines for treatment of sexually transmitted disease. *Morbidity and Mortality Weekly Report, 55*(11).

Gabbe, S. G., Niebyl, J. R., & Simpson, J. L. (2007). *Obstetrics: Normal and problem pregnancies* (5th ed.). Philadelphia, PA: Churchill Livingstone.

Gibbs, R., Karlan, B., Haney, A., & Nygaard, I. (2008). *Danforth's obstetrics and gynecology* (10th ed.). Philadelphia, PA: Williams, Wilkins, and Wolters.

Institute of Medicine (IOM). (2009). *Weight gain during pregnancy: Reexamining the guidelines.* Washington, DC: Author.

Lowdermilk, D., & Perry, S. (2007). *Maternity and women's health* (9th ed.). Philadelphia, PA: Mosby Elsevier.

Seidel, H., Ball, J., Dains, J., & Benedict, W. (2006). *Mosby's guide to physical examination* (6th ed.). St. Louis, MO: Mosby.

Tharpe, N., & Farley, C. (2009). *Clinical practice guidelines for midwifery and women's health* (3rd ed.). Sudbury, MA: Jones and Bartlett.

4

Professional Issues

Beth M. Kelsey

Select one best answer to the following questions.

1. The research method that uses a subjective approach to describe life experiences and give them meaning is:

   a. Correlational
   b. Qualitative
   c. Quasi-experimental
   d. Quantitative

2. A research study is designed to determine if providing information about contraceptive methods to high school students will reduce the number of pregnancies that occur prior to graduation. The 9th grade class will be provided with information on contraceptive methods, and the 10th grade class will not be given any information. The number of pregnancies that occur prior to graduation in both classes will be compared. The dependent variable in this study is:

   a. Contraceptive information
   b. Number of pregnancies
   c. The 9th grade class
   d. The 10th grade class

3. One measure of central tendency is the median. The median of the following values (9,10,10,12,15,16,18) is:

   a. 10
   b. 12
   c. 14
   d. 15

4. The statement that predicts the expected relationship between two or more variables in a study is the:

   a. Analysis of variance
   b. Level of significance
   c. Hypothesis
   d. Research design

5. You are reading a research study that was designed to measure the occurrence of postpartum depression in adolescent mothers. After reading the study, you question whether the instrument used in the study was actually able to measure postpartum depression in adolescent mothers. What is it about the study that you are questioning?

   a. Reliability
   b. Generalization
   c. Significance
   d. Validity

6. In which of the following studies would a longitudinal design be most appropriate?

   a. Comparison of factors associated with condom use of high school freshmen, sophomores, juniors, and seniors
   b. Determining the extent to which risk factors predict fractures in older women
   c. Determining why women discontinue oral contraceptives within the first 3 months of use
   d. Determining an organization's status related to the problem of patient falls

7. The "reasonable person standard" is used to describe one of the components necessary for:

   a. Breach of duty
   b. Informed consent
   c. Intentional torts
   d. Standards of practice

8. A 28-year-old woman recently had a hysterectomy for invasive cervical cancer. She has filed a malpractice suit against the healthcare provider who performed her Pap test 3 years ago. The Pap test result showed a high-grade lesion. Pap tests prior to that were normal. In accordance with the clinic's protocol, three attempts were made to contact the patient. The third attempt was sent by certified mail. This letter came back showing that the patient had moved leaving no forwarding address. Which element, that must be proved by the patient for a malpractice suit based on negligence, is absent?

   a. Duty
   b. Breach of duty
   c. Actual damages
   d. Causation

9. A malpractice claim is made against a nurse practitioner. The incident related to the claim occurred 3 years ago. Which of the following types of liability policies would cover this claim?

   a. Claims made coverage policy in effect at the time of the incident that lapsed 1 year ago
   b. Claims made policy purchased in the current year with tail coverage
   c. Occurrence-based coverage policy in effect at the time of the incident that lapsed 2 years ago
   d. Occurrence-based coverage policy that was purchased in the past year

10. Legal scope of practice for the advanced practice nurse is defined by:

    a. National certification organizations
    b. National advanced practice nursing organizations
    c. School of nursing accreditation organizations
    d. State boards of nursing

11. Providing the patient information on the benefits and risks of a treatment and alternatives so she can make an informed decision most clearly addresses the ethical principles of:

    a. Beneficence and respect for autonomy
    b. Fidelity and veracity
    c. Nonmaleficence and fidelity
    d. Privacy and formal justice

12. Which of the following statements is correct related to standards of care?

    a. Following standards of care assures that the advanced practice nurse will not be sued for malpractice
    b. The advanced practice nurse may be held to the same standard of care as a physician
    c. Your state board of nursing is responsible for notifying you of changes in standards of care
    d. Where you live does not have any significance when determining if standards of care were followed

13. Using random sampling to choose subjects for a study is one method used to promote:

    a. Generalizability
    b. Reliability

c.   Triangulation
d.   Validity

14. The major role of an institutional review board (IRB) is to:

a.   Assure the study is feasible in terms
of time and costs
b.   Assure the rights of human subjects
are being protected
c.   Critique the proposal and provide
suggestions to improve the design
d.   Evaluate the credentials of the in-
vestigators of the proposed study

◻ ANSWERS AND RATIONALE

1. **(b)** Qualitative research methods
use a systematic, subjective approach
to describe life experiences and give
them meaning. This type of research
is conducted to describe and promote
understanding of human experiences
such as pain, loss, powerlessness, and
caring. Quantitative research uses a formal, objective, and systematic process
in which numerical data are utilized to
obtain information, describe variables,
examine relationships between variables, and determine cause and effect.
Correlational and quasi-experimental
research are both types of quantitative research (Boswell & Cannon, pp.
164–166; Schmidt & Brown, p. 14).

2. **(b)** The dependent variable in a study
is the response, behavior, or outcome
that is predicted or explained in research. Changes in the dependent
variable (number of pregnancies) are
presumed to be caused by the inde-
pendent variable (contraceptive information). The 9th grade class is the
experimental group and the 10th grade
class is the control group (Boswell &
Cannon, pp. 83, 276–277; Schmidt &
Brown, p. 124).

3. **(b)** The median is the score or number
at the exact center of a group of numbers. Three numbers fall on either side

of 12 so it is the median value. Other
measures of central tendency include
the mean, the mode, and standard
deviation (Boswell & Cannon, p. 273;
Schmidt & Brown, pp. 259–260).

4. **(c)** The hypothesis is a formal statement of the expected relationship
between two or more variables in a
specified population. The hypothesis
in the study described in question # 2
might be that providing contraceptive
information to high school students in
the ninth grade will reduce the number of pregnancies that occur prior to
graduation by 50% (Boswell & Cannon,
pp. 294–295; Schmidt & Brown, p. 64).

5. **(d)** A valid instrument measures the
construct that it is intended to measure. Reliability is concerned with how
consistently an instrument measures
the concept of interest. Generalization
extends the implications of the findings
from the sample studied to the larger
population. Significance can either refer to results that are in keeping with
those identified by the researcher, or
the statistically determined level of
significance (Boswell & Cannon, p. 237;
Schmidt & Brown, pp. 197–200).

6. **(b)** Longitudinal study design—also
known as a prospective study design—
is used to gather data about subjects at
more than one point in time. This type
of design is useful when the researcher
has identified presumed causes and
then follows subjects into the future
to determine if hypothesized effects
actually occur. An example is the obser-
vational component of the Women's
Health Initiative. Postmenopausal
women were followed over time to
determine the extent to which known
risk factors predict heart disease, cancer, and fractures in older women.
The comparison of factors associated
with condom use among the different
classes of high school students might
be done with a cross-sectional design.

The researcher looking at why women discontinue oral contraceptives within the first 3 months of use might conduct a retrospective study asking women to recall their reasons for discontinuation. An organization could use a retrospective chart audit to determine number of patient falls as well as looking for causative factors (Schmidt & Brown, pp. 135–139).

7. **(b)** The "reasonable person standard" applies to informed consent. Whether a patient's consent to a procedure was informed depends on whether the healthcare provider who performed the procedure disclosed all of the facts, risks, and alternatives that a reasonable person would need to make a decision (Hamric, Spross, & Hanson, p. 547; Buppert, p. 271–272).

8. **(b)** Negligence is the failure to act in a reasonable way as a healthcare provider. For a negligence malpractice suit to be valid there must be a duty of care, breach of providing that care within accepted standards, injury to the patient, and demonstrated causation that the injury was caused by the healthcare provider. Breach of duty means that the healthcare provider failed to perform a duty that she had to the patient. In this situation, the duty is to inform a patient of the abnormal results of a Pap test. The healthcare provider followed the clinic's protocol and made three attempts to contact the patient, including a certified letter that was returned indicating that the patient had moved and left no forwarding address. This would generally be considered to have met the accepted standard of care and the duty of the healthcare provider. Actual damages would be the hysterectomy and loss of fertility. Not having the Pap test results may have delayed early treatment that might have been less extensive, preserving the uterus (Hamric, Spross, & Hanson, pp. 618–619).

9. **(c)** An occurrence-based policy provides coverage for any incident that occurred during the time the policy was in effect. Claims made policies cover the individual for any suit filed while the policy is in effect. Tail coverage extends claims made coverage into the future to cover claims filed after the basic claims coverage period (Buppert, p. 264; Hamric, Spross, & Hanson, pp. 619–620).

10. **(d)** Scope of practice refers to the legal authority granted to a profession to provide healthcare services. For advanced practice nurses, scope of practice is most closely tied to state board of nursing statutes or regulations defined by nurse practice acts (Buppert, pp. 37–38).

11. **(a)** Respect for autonomy reflects the duty to respect others' personal liberty and individual values, beliefs, and choices. Beneficence refers to the duty to do good and prevent or remove harm. Nonmaleficence is the duty not to inflict harm, and fidelity is the duty to honor commitments. Veracity refers to the duty to tell the truth and not to deceive others (Hamric, Spross, & Hanson, p. 324).

12. **(b)** The standard of care is determined by asking what a qualified healthcare provider in the same geographic area, in the same general type of practice, in a similar situation would do. If the advanced practice nurse is providing care that is typically provided by a physician in her geographic area, she may be held to the same standard of care as the physician. The healthcare professional is responsible for keeping up to date with standards of care for specific diseases and for healthcare maintenance through continuing education, reading professional journals, and monitoring government and professional organization-generated guidelines (Buppert, pp. 267–268).

13. **(a)** Generalizability refers to the extent to which research findings from a study can be inferred from a sample population to the population at large. Random sampling involves processes to assure that each element of the population has an equal chance of being in the sample. Using random sampling reduces the threat of selection bias and should result in a more representative sample. Finding that multiple studies have obtained similar results also increases the extent to which one can generalize the findings to a wider population (Boswell & Cannon, pp. 126, 341; Schmidt & Brown, p. 59, 215–217).

14. **(b)** The major role of an institutional review board (IRB) is to evaluate the ethical considerations related to a proposed or ongoing research study in order to protect human subjects (Boswell & Cannon, p. 342; Schmidt & Brown, pp. 46–47).

◻ REFERENCES

Boswell, C., & Cannon, S. (2007). *Introduction to nursing research: Incorporating evidence-based practice.* Sudbury, MA: Jones and Bartlett.

Buppert, C. (2008). *Nurse practitioner's business practice and legal guide* (3rd ed.). Sudbury, MA: Jones and Bartlett.

Hamric, A., Spross, J., & Hanson, C. (2009). *Advanced practice nursing: An integrative approach* (4th ed.). St. Louis, MO: Saunders.

Schmidt, N., & Brown, J. (2009). *Evidence-based practice for nurses: Appraisal and application of research.* Sudbury, MA: Jones and Bartlett.

Index

Notes

Notes

Notes

Notes

Notes

Notes

Notes

Notes

Notes

Notes